A TREATISE

ON

DISEASES OF THE EYE;

FOR THE USE OF

GENERAL PRACTITIONERS.

BY

H. C. ANGELL, M.D.,

OPHTHALMIC SURGEON TO THE BOSTON HOMŒOPATHIC MEDICAL DISPENSARY.

BOSTON:

JAMES CAMPBELL, PUBLISHER,

18, Tremont Street, Museum Building.

1870.

CAMBRIDGE:
PRESS OF JOHN WILSON AND SON.

THIS BOOK IS DEDICATED

TO

ROBERT ELLIS DUDGEON,

M.D., L.R.C.S. EDIN., ETC., ETC.,

Of London, England,

AS A TRIBUTE OF RESPECT FOR HIS WORTH AS AN AUTHOR AND AS A PHYSICIAN.

PREFACE.

My readers are requested to bear in mind that this work is written, not for specialists, but for homœopathic physicians in general practice — for those too busied with the whole, to devote a great amount of time to any one part of medicine and surgery. The endeavor has been, to treat the subjects embraced, clearly and concisely, in the hope of presenting a volume attractive enough, and small enough, to induce the busiest to give it some attention. That there is need of works of this kind in our school is, I presume, unquestioned; and some of the reasons why this need has been permitted to exist so long, are given very frankly in the large treatise of Bæhr, translated by Hempel. The author remarks, in speaking of our neglect of ophthalmic practice, that " we are yet too much upon the defensive towards our professional opponents to enjoy the privilege of exclusively cultivating a department that requires extraordinary manual dexterity." He then relates the nature of other obstacles, chiefly those arising from a lack of hospitals and clinical teaching, and finally remarks that, if they were removed, "an oculist would still have a great many difficulties to contend with, which are inherent in our materia medica. We confess, without hesitation," he adds, "that there is no section of our materia medica less useful and less adapted to homœopathic treatment, than the symptoms referring to diseases of the eye." All these obstacles are, however, soon to be swept away. Hospitals are established and being established all over the country; these will give us an opportunity for instruction and improvement in special branches, and with this increased interest in special departments, will come, in due time, its legitimate fruit — a separate and distinct literature for each important class of diseases.

In the preparation of this work, I have had the advantage of copious notes taken during a somewhat prolonged attendance at the European clinics; and I have availed myself without hesitation, also, of the privilege of taking and appropriating whatever I have found desirable in the standard or periodical works devoted to ophthalmology.

CONTENTS.

CHAPTER VI.

THE CORNEA AND SCLEROTICA.

CHAPTER VII.

THE IRIS.

CHAPTER VIII.

THE CHOROID AND VITREOUS.

CHAPTER IX.

GLAUCOMA.

CHAPTER X.

THE RETINA AND OPTIC NERVE.

CHAPTER XI.

AMBLYOPIA.

CHAPTER XII.

THE CRYSTALLINE LENS.

CHAPTER XIII.

SPECTACLES — ARTIFICIAL EYES.

CHAPTER XIV.

THE MUSCLES OF THE EYE.

CHAPTER XV.

THE EYELIDS.

CHAPTER XVI.

THE LACHRYMAL APPARATUS.

CHAPTER XVII.

CHAPTER XVIII.

CHAPTER XIX.

CHAPTER XX.

CHAPTER XI.

PAGE

AMBLYOPIA.

CHAPTER XII.

THE CRYSTALLINE LENS.

CHAPTER XIII.

SPECTACLES — ARTIFICIAL EYES.

CHAPTER XIV.

THE MUSCLES OF THE EYE.

CHAPTER XV.

THE EYELIDS.

CHAPTER XVI.

THE LACHRYMAL APPARATUS.

CHAPTER XVII.

CHAPTER XVIII.

CHAPTER XIX.

CHAPTER XX.

DISEASES OF THE EYE.

CHAPTER I.

BRIEF SKETCH OF THE RISE AND PROGRESS OF OPHTHALMIC SURGERY.

It appears that the ancient Egyptians were the first to divide the practice of medicine and surgery into distinct departments, and that in those days there were practitioners who devoted themselves especially to the study and treatment of diseases of the eye and ear. That no progress of consequence was made in medicine at that epoch is to be attributed to the primitive condition of anatomy and pathology, and to the circumstance that whatever knowledge of this kind existed was regarded as the exclusive property of its possessor, to be left like an heirloom to his family or his successor.

The Arabians, Greeks, and Romans possessed considerable information in regard to diseases of the eye; and Celsus, in the first century, wrote accurately on diseases of the eyelids, described pterygium, and an operation for its removal not unlike that practised at the present day.

After this we hear little of disease of the eye, until the beginning of the eighteenth century; and even as late as this, oculists were but itinerant quacks and lecturers, who trumpeted their fame at fairs, in front of the booths in which they practised. There were female oculists also in those days. An author of that time says, "About five years since, I saw a woman in Holborn, by King's Gate, that had a dissolution of vitreous humor in the right eye, a narrowness of the inward chamber and immobility of the pupil, and half was dilated. The crystalline was opaque and shrunk in its bigness, pressed against the pupil and was of whitish-gray, by reason of the fibrous parts of its crooked and contracted segments, so that she could not perceive any light with that eye. She asked me if I could do her any good; I told her there was no hope, for she could not see the least glimmering because her cataract was accompanied with a gutta serena which was perfect. She told me that Mrs. Jones, a famous woman for couching of cataracts, would have couched her some years before." The same author writes of the "Cataplexia of the eye which Hippocrates speaks of," and goes on in this remarkable way: "Some call this the conick movement which is the parrexis or helcosis and abruption precision, or ulceration and solution of the continuity of the optic nerve, caused from a stroke wound or fall of humors or apostimation." He says further that the "Syntosis of Galen or the syntomosis is a collaption, compression, flabbiness of said nerve, which is affected by dryness," and so on. Some of the remedies in use only one hundred and fifty years ago are equally remarkable. A scarificator was made of beards of barley tied into a little brush. Applications in common use were vipers' fat, gall of the eel and pike, a mixture of ants and honey, and applications of a less delicate nature. As original and curious as any, was the insertion in the eye of a living louse, of which it was affirmed, probably with good reason, that "it tickleth and pricketh and rendereth the eye moist and rheumatic."

Towards the middle of the last century the attention of the profession in Germany began to be directed particularly towards the study of ophthalmology, and this awakened interest finally led, in 1773, to the foundation at Vienna, in connection with the University, of a department of ophthalmology. This school became famous for its successful and distinguished teachers, and in this respect flourished without a rival up to a very recent period. Scarpa's excellent treatise on Diseases of the Eye was published in 1801, that of Beer in 1815, Guthrie's, the first complete work in English, and long a standard in this country, in 1823. Then followed the standard works of Lawrence, Tyrrell, and McKenzie, and in Germany those of Rozas, Juenken, and Arlt.

About the year 1840, Dieffenbach, of Berlin first practised his operation for the cure of strabismus, the success of which gave an impulse to the study of the physiology and pathology of the muscles of the eyeball, and has resulted in the exhaustive researches on this subject of the two Graefes and others.

We come now to the year 1851, the date of the discovery of the ophthalmoscope. From the very earliest times the luminosity of the eye, especially in the cat and the dog, had been observed, and had been regarded by the people with superstitious awe. In the year 1704 Méry saw the retinal vessels in the eye of a cat under water, but not until some years later was the cause of this luminosity properly referred to light received into the eye from without. Cumming, in 1846, came very near depriving Helmholtz of the honor of his great discovery, and Reute, who improved the ophthalmoscope in 1852 and rendered it practical, may be fairly said to divide the honor of its invention with Helmholtz.

Since the discovery of this instrument the progress of ophthalmology in all its branches has been not only rapid beyond precedent, but more rapid than the most sanguine could have hoped for. It is impossible here to more than allude to some of these great advances and their results. Recognition and accurate description of the different diseases of the optic nerve and retina and their frequent connection with affection of the brain, heart, and kidney; diagnosis of diseases of the choroid and vitreous; classification of opacities of the lens giving rise to variety and improvement in operations for cataract; the operation of iridectomy, rendering glaucoma a curable disease; improved methods of making artificial pupil; rational surgical treatment of disorders of the lachrymal apparatus; demonstration of the laws of refraction and accommodation of the eye, which has been of incalculable value in the diagnosis and treatment of a large class of cases where imperfect vision is a prominent symptom; the diagnosis and cure of astigmatism; the progress in entoptics; the detection of cysticerci in the eye; the treatment of conical cornea; the use of the compressive bandage; the introduction of the use of atropine and the calabar bean; the invention of the aut-ophthalmoscope whereby we may examine at our leisure the fundus of our own eyes and "see oursel's as others see us"; the more cautious and less indiscriminate use of caustics, and the almost entire abolition of the so-called heroic antiphlogistic measures in disease of the eye, — these and many other improvements in diagnosis and treatment, which I do not mention even by name, are the results of the marvellous impulse given to the study of disease of the eye by the discovery of the ophthalmoscope.

CHAPTER II.

EXAMINATION OF THE EYES.

OBJECTIVE EXAMINATION.

AFTER a glance at the exterior aspect of the lids, their margin, the cilia, the general appearance of the eyeball as to position or prominence, we may turn our attention to the different tunics of the globe which permit of examination from without. For this purpose a good light is necessary, and the best, generally speaking, is that which falls obliquely on the eye of the patient from a very near window. A still stronger light may be had, when necessary, by *lateral illumination*, as explained in the chapter on the Ophthalmoscope. If we suspect a foreign body, if conjunctivitis with discharge be present, if the lids seem thickened, if any sensation is complained of beneath the upper lid, if there is enlargement of the mucous papillæ of the lower lid, the upper lid should be reversed. This proceeding requires but a moment, can never do harm, and may often give us at once the key to the difficulty.

To reverse the upper lid it is merely necessary to raise it slightly with the thumb of the left hand, then seizing firmly the central cilia and edge of the tarsus between the forefinger and thumb of the right hand, the lid is pulled slightly downward and away from the eyeball, and while the patient is requested to look downward, at this instant the lid is tilted over the point of the left thumb, which is used as a fulcrum. If necessary, a probe may be used as a fulcrum, placing it half an inch above the margin of the lid and parallel with it. The signification of the various kinds of redness of the eye is noticed under simple conjunctivitis. The surface of the cornea should be carefully scrutinized for delicate opacity, ulceration, abrasion, or unevenness.

A few weeks since a young lady called for me to aid her in the selection of suitable glasses. She did not see well at a distance. I expected to find, upon examination, that she was either myopic or hypermetropic. To my surprise there was neither myopia, hypermetropia, or astigmatism present. Nor could I find any abnormal condition of the eye whatever. I thought of old opacity of the cornea, but did not find it. After learning, however, that in childhood she had suffered from an affection which was undoubtedly a purulent ophthalmia, I felt positive that the cornea must be at fault. On taking her again into a darkened room, and re-examining the surface of the cornea by oblique illumination, *and comparing her eyes* under the strong light with those of her companion, I discovered a delicate cloudiness in both corneæ. Without the aid of lateral illumination and the comparison with the perfect cornea of a normal eye, the haziness would have escaped detection.

The size of the pupil, its form, its mobility, and the color of the iris should be noted. The mobility may be tested by permitting the eye to be closed and then raising the upper lid gently with the thumb, observing the reduction in the size of the pupil as the light strikes the eye, or, by shading the opened eye with the hand, then removing the hand suddenly. In either of these experiments the eye not under examination must be closed, to avoid sympathetic influence between the two. If the pupil is sluggish in movement, or does not look exactly circular, or if the iris is at all discolored, we should drop into the eye a solution of atropine (one or two grains to the ounce of water), in order to determine whether there is adhesion between the posterior surface of the iris and the anterior surface of the capsule of the lens. If adhesions exist the enlarged pupil will be irregular in form. It is sometimes necessary to use a solution of atropine stronger than this, of four or six grains to the ounce, when the iris is diseased, in order to affect the size of the pupil sufficiently. See article on Mydriasis. The appearance of the surface of the iris may be abnormal as to color, texture, plastic deposits, and condylomata. The significance of these objective examinations and their details will be found when we come to speak of the diseases of the various structures of the eye.

Tension or *hardness* of the eyeball is to be noted in order to determine the degree of intra-ocular pressure. It is determined by gentle pressure through the closed lids upon the eyeball with the forefinger. The two eyes may be compared, or a sound eye with the diseased one, in order to fix the degree of hardness or softness with more accuracy. Signs to denote the amount of intra-ocular pressure are sometimes used. Thus: T. 1, T. 2, T. 3: indicate first degree or slight, second degree or considerable, third degree or extreme tension (hardness) of the ball; while Tn., T? indicate tension normal, tension doubtful. The same letter and figures preceded by the sign minus mean reduced tension or softness of the globe. Thus: —T. 1, first degree of reduced tension.

The mobility of the eye is to be tested by requesting the patient to follow the finger, which is moved in various directions, in order to detect paralysis of any muscle, or the finger may be moved towards the eyes as directed under muscular asthenopia, to determine the strength of the recti interni muscles.

SUBJECTIVE EXAMINATION.

THE PAIN.

The nature, seat, and severity of the pain complained of by the patient is of importance as an aid to diagnosis and *a fortiori* to the selection of appropriate remedies. A dull pain in and around the eyeball, with a sensation of heat, the pain very much increased by using the eye, points to asthenopia. Smarting and burning, and a sensation as if sand were in the eye, indicates a conjunctivitis. Severe pain with photophobia and lachrymation denotes sensitiveness of the ciliary nerves, as in deep-seated conjunctivitis, corneitis, iritis, or any inflammation affecting the ciliary region, at the junction of the cornea and sclerotica. Deep-seated pain in the eye, or just above it, recurring periodically, accompanied by dimness of vision, is to be seriously regarded, and is characteristic of beginning glaucoma.

The severity of the pain, however, is not alone a safe criterion by which to judge the gravity or slightness of an affection of the eye. When present, it helps us to determine the nature of the disease, but it may be absent sometimes in the most serious cases, such for instance as glaucoma, amaurosis, or choroiditis.

Photophobia, with no pain, or appearances of inflammation externally, indicates hyperæthesia retinæ — too great a sensibility of the retina. Retinitis, by itself, is a rare disease, and would be characterized by a want of sensibility and the necessity of a strong light to see distinctly.

THE STATE OF THE VISION.

The visual power of a diseased eye is an important diagnostic point to determine. This will be best investigated by the use of the test types annexed to this volume. If the patient reads No. 1 or 2 readily, and also the letters of No. 12, 15, or 20, at twelve, fifteen, or twenty feet respectively, with the naked eye or by the help of suitable spectacles, his sight is perfect. His visual power = 1. Good sight for a few moments followed by confusion of vision, suggests asthenopia. Rapid diminution of vision as objects recede from the eye, points to myopia. Lack of clearness in regarding objects near and distant, indicates hypermetropia. Defective sight for near objects and normal vision for distance, is characteristic of presbyopia. Cloudiness of sight, improved towards night and in dull weather, suggests cataract. If "spectacles never did any good" we think of astigmatism; then amblyopia, and serious internal disease of the eye will be thought of if glasses have recently ceased to be of use. If the patient cannot see the largest sized letters, he may be able to count fingers held quite near the eye Failing in this he may distinguish between light and darkness. Seat him before a window, and then interpose between his eyes and the light some dark object of sufficient size; or, a still better test, because it admits of measurement, is to take the patient into a room from which daylight is wholly excluded. He may be able to point in the direction of the lamplight, even if it is quite dim; or he may be able to discern it only when it is very brilliant, or he may not be able to see it at all. If he cannot tell with certainty, standing near the light whether we shade it from him or whether it shines full in his face, there is no vision to be improved, and no restoration of sight is possible. In these experiments, if one eye alone is being tested, cover the other with the folded handkerchief so as to exclude all sight from it. A healthy eye will readily distinguish light from darkness with the lids firmly closed.

THE FIELD OF VISION.

The extent of the field of vision may be determined by directing the patient to look steadily at one finger held before his eye at a distance of eighteen or twenty inches. We then move our other hand about at a distance of two feet below, above, and on each side, from the finger towards which the patient is steadily to look, noting whether he sees the hand or can count the fingers. The finger which we hold up is at the centre of the visual field, and it may be necessary to bring the other hand very near to this before it can be seen. A few weeks since I found the field of vision so much narrowed in a case of *retinitis pigmentosa* that the patient could not distinguish an object moving until it came within an inch or an inch and a half of the centre of the field; showing that only a part even of the yellow spot itself retained its normal function. A normal eye will distinguish an object moving at a distance of from two to three feet from the central point of vision. The field of vision may be mapped out when great accuracy is desirable. Put the patient before a blackboard, at the distance of fifteen inches; make a dot for him to fix the eye on; then approach a piece of chalk in a long black handle from different directions, recording always the point where the chalk is first perceived by a dot; afterwards unite these dots by a continuous line, and the boundaries of the field of vision are sketched.

DIPLOPIA.

Double images occur in paralytic strabismus, and frequently after an operation for the cure of concomitant strabismus. Monocular diplopia is a result of irregular refraction from abnormal curvature of the cornea or lens, of mal-position or dislocation of the lens, of inequalities of the corneal surface from old cicatrices, or of bands of membrane stretched across the area of the pupil. We may readily produce double images by holding a convex lens of medium strength partly before one eye so that we may look through it and not through it at the same time, at objects across the room.

IMPLEMENTS AND INSTRUMENTS.

TRIAL GLASSES.

Complete sets of trial glasses, or spectacles, are necessary for those who propose to prescribe suitable glasses for the various optical defects. The selection of proper glasses for patients is a very important and responsible duty, and should not be undertaken unless the practitioner is disposed to give sufficient attention to it to do it in a scientific manner. Let the reprehensible, hap-hazard selection of glasses be left to the itinerant vender and optician. The proper glass having been determined, its number and kind are to be written out and presented by the patient to a respectable optician. A complete outfit of trial glasses comprising the convex and concave, spherical and cylindrical, the prismatic and the colored, will amount to some two hundred, or the equivalent of a hundred pairs of spectacles. To such as do not propose a more or less complete equipment for the above purpose, I would suggest a few glasses merely as an aid in diagnosis.

Weak convex lenses, of 30, 40, and 50 inch focus, will help to determine a hypermetropia, or a beginning presbyopia. If the patient sees No. 20 at twenty feet as well with as without, or better with than without either of the glasses, he is hypermetropic. In beginning presbyopia the same glasses should aid in reading the No. 1 print. Ordinary concave glasses will aid in the differential diagnosis of a slight myopia and hypermetropia. Through concaves of 30, 40, or 50 inch focus, a myope should see distant objects more clearly. The same spherical convex or concave glasses will aid in determining an astigmatism, in connection with the metallic plate and slit. A slip of colored glass will be useful in testing double images, and a few prisms are necessary to measure the strength of the ocular muscles, and to aid in curing some forms of strabismus.

The ophthalmoscope is very useful, and perhaps ought now to be considered indispensable to the general practitioner. Very necessary also are a pair of silver lid elevators for the purpose chiefly of elevating the eyelids of unruly children, and for the extraction of foreign bodies imbedded in the cornea, a wire speculum self-adjusting, a fine needle and a delicate spatula, spud or grooved needle, and a pair of delicate forceps for steadying the eyeball in case this is necessary. The Snellen eye-lid tourniquet is an almost indispensable aid in removing cysts of the lids.

BANDAGING THE EYE.

The ordinary bandage may consist of a piece of linen about ten inches long by two and a quarter inches in width, with a piece of broad tape at either end to pass around the head, and tie. A third tape may pass over the top of the head to assist in holding the bandage in place when necessary. Before applying, a bit of linen and a little charpie should be placed over the closed eye.

The compress bandage should be one and three-quarters yards in length and about one and a half inches in width, and made of linen, or, still better, fine elastic flannel. To apply it, commence above the affected eye, pass it across the forehead to the opposite side, above the ear, to the back of the head, below the ear, then up across the bit of linen and charpie upon the affected eye, and pin it securely to the first portion upon the forehead.

CHAPTER III.

THE OPHTHALMOSCOPE.

In order to see into the interior of an eye, it is necessary first of all that the interior should be lighted up. The old notion that an eye under certain nervous conditions becomes luminous from within is not correct. It can be illuminated only by light from without. The second condition necessary is, that, having thrown rays of light into the eye under examination, we should place our own eye in such a position relative to the one illuminated, as to catch the reflection of the rays of light which we have thrown in. These two conditions are absolutely necessary, and any further ones merely add to the convenience of examination or render our examination more accurate. With a bit of common window-glass we can fulfil these two conditions. Seat the patient in a darkened room with a lighted lamp by his side, the flame about on a level with the eye to be examined. With this fragment of glass held in front of the pupil and quite near the eye under examination, throw the rays of light from the lamp directly into his eye. This fulfils the first condition. The eye is illuminated. Now put your own eye behind the glass directly opposite that of the patient, and it will catch the return rays passing from his eye through the glass into yours, and you will see the entrance of the optic nerve, or optic disc as it is termed, and the vessels of the retina passing over and away from it. The fragment of glass is in reality an ophthalmoscope, and all ophthalmoscopes are merely modifications of this, and do not differ from it in principle. It has been found more convenient, however, to substitute for the plane glass a concave mirror * with a small hole at its centre for the eye of the observer. A concave mirror reflects more light into the eye, and hence renders the details of the fundus more distinct. To the same end also it has been found serviceable in practice to hold immediately before the observed eye with the left hand, a convex glass of about two-inch focus. This convex lens enlarges the field of vision; and, although we get an inverted image, on the whole it facilitates an examination so much as to render its use almost indispensable in the examination of the deeper struc-

* Sometimes, a plane or even a slightly convex mirror is preferred.

tures of the eye. There are some forty or fifty different kinds of ophthalmoscopes in use. The one most common, and the one I generally use, is that of Liebreich. It consists of a metallic mirror slightly concave, about an inch and an eighth in diameter, set in a metallic frame, with a handle which pushes into itself so as to be no more than two inches in length when not in use, and convenient for the pocket. In the centre of the mirror is an aperture one-eighth of an inch in diameter, and attached to the frame of the mirror is a hinged bracket to hold a small convex or concave lens, to assist the eye of the observer if necessary. The object glass or convex lens is rather larger than the mirror, of about two-inch focus, and may be set also in a metallic frame with a short handle. A very interesting form of instrument is the binocular ophthalmoscope, so constructed that by means of prisms we are enabled to use both eyes at once in an examination. Through this we obtain a stereoscopic view of the fundus, all its parts being brought into relief. We can readily determine any change of surface on the optic disc, small excavations or a slight prominence. It is easier with this instrument also to determine the relative positions of opacities in the vitreous humor or extravasations in the retina or choroid. Attractive, however, as the binocular ophthalmoscope seems to be, I find that in practice I seldom use it. It is large, cumbersome, and heavy, and requires more time for its proper use, and ordinarily, therefore, its advantages do not in practice appear to be of sufficient importance to compel its employment. For many difficult cases it is, however, almost indispensable.

Another, the aut-ophthalmoscope, is so arranged that, by an ingenious combination of mirrors, one may look with his right eye directly into his left, or *vice versa.* There are also fixed ophthalmoscopes, large and heavy, but useful in the class-room, and for sketching the appearance of the fundus.

HOW TO USE THE OPHTHALMOSCOPE.

In the beginning, in order to learn to use the ophthalmoscope, it is best to examine a number of healthy eyes. It is advisable also to dilate the pupil with a weak solution of atropine, — one grain to ten or twelve ounces of water, — which will so enlarge the field of vision as to make the examination more interesting and instructive. The advantage of a weak solution is that its effect on the pupil vanishes within about twenty-four hours. A stronger solution will act more quickly, but will not pass off in two or three days, or perhaps a week. The instillation of atropine does no permanent harm, but while the pupil is under its influence, being widely dilated, a strong light is somewhat dazzling and vision is more or less impaired for near objects. It must be remembered that if we use the convex object glass we get an *indirect* or *inverted* picture of the fundus, and without the interposition of the object glass we get a *direct* or *upright image*. Having seated our patient in a room from which daylight is completely excluded with a good steady light at his left side, we take up the mirror in the right hand, put it close to our own eye and our eye to the aperture, and on a line with the eye to be examined, and distant from it perhaps eight to twelve inches. Turning the mirror slightly towards the lamp, we readily illuminate the eye of the patient. Already we have learned something, because all eyes cannot be illuminated, — an opaque lens, for instance, prevents it. Now, hold with the left hand the convex object glass before the illuminated eye, at the distance of an inch and a half or two inches, directing the patient to look in the direction of our left ear when we are to examine his left eye, and our right ear when we direct our attention to his right eye, — in other words, directing that the eye under examination shall be turned slightly inwards so as to bring the optic nerve directly opposite or behind the pupil. To examine the region of the macula lutea the patient should look straight forward, directly at the eyes of the observer. It will be recognized as a spot slightly darker in color, with no vessels running over it. Having illuminated the fundus of the eye with the mirror in the right hand, we must be careful not to change its position while we are adjusting the convex glass held in the left hand, otherwise we shall fail to see the interior of the eye from lack of light. Until the beginner learns to use the hands independently of each other, he may expect to trace one or more failures to a well-intentioned illumination of a button-hole of his patient's coat.

If the patient is myopic we gain a more distinct view by approaching our own eye a little, and if he is hypermetropic we see better by increasing, slightly, the distance between our eye and his. If our own eye is presbyopic or hypermetropic we may also find it advantageous to use in the hinged bracket behind the mirror one of the little convex glasses of eight or ten-inch focus which belongs to the ophthalmoscope. The convex glasses will also be found serviceable if the eye of the patient is hypermetropic.

In the *direct examination* without the object glass in the left hand, if we desire to examine the disc or fundus, we must approach our eye very near to that of the patient; but to simply test the transparency of the media, — the lens or humors, — we place our own eye at a distance of fifteen or eighteen inches from the eye under observation.

The appearance of the fundus of the normal eye differs considerably in different individuals. The fundus of the eye of a light-complexioned person is light-red, while that of a dark-complexioned one is dark-red, owing to an abundance of pigment in the choroid. In the former, the epithelial layer of the choroid being less pigmented, we may see many of the vessels of the choroid through it, which gives the fundus a striated appearance. In very dark eyes the choroidal vessels are invisible.

The disc or optic nerve entrance appears generally, to me, of a slightly yellowish-grayish pink. In dark eyes more white and glistening, in light eyes more rosy in color. It is usually circular in form, but in astigmatism often has the appearance of being oval when it really is circular.* Its edge is sharply de-

---

* Suppose, for instance, a case of astigmatism where the cornea is too convex in the vertical meridian. The optic disc appears oval in a vertical direction if we make a direct examination. In *indirect examination* it will appear *oval in a horizontal direction.* The reason of this is plain. Our convex glass makes objects appear larger if held near them, but if removed from the object beyond its focus (about two inches) we have an image inverted and reduced in size. Now in a case like the above, the eye lends the greater refracting power to the glass in a vertical direction, and the inverted and reduced image will, of course, be reduced most in the direction of the greatest refractive power. The convexity of the glass and the cornea combined being greater in the vertical line, the inverted image of the disc is reduced most in this direction. Hence it appears oval horizontally.

fined, and near it may be seen occasionally a slight crescentic line of pigment. The face of the disc is more pinkish at its inner half, and where the retinal vessels emerge from it.

The *retinal vessels* run principally upward and downward, an artery, known by its light color, and two veins running in each direction. The retina itself, in a healthy state, is transparent, and cannot be seen. Exceptionally in very dark eyes, it may be detected as a gray film, in the immediate vicinity of the disc. The *physiological excavation*, not unfrequently noticed in the healthy nerve disc, is spoken of in connection with pathological excavations in the remarks on atrophy of the optic nerve or amaurosis. *Venous pulsation* may sometimes be observed in the healthy eye. It is to be looked for in that part of the retinal vein between the centre of the nerve disc and its edges. It may be produced by gentle pressure on the ball of the eye with the finger. Similar arterial pulsation indicates intraocular pressure, and is not found in the healthy eye.

The ophthalmoscopic appearance of *the diseased eye* is spoken of in connection with the various affections, which demand its aid for their diagnosis and intelligent treatment. I may remark here, however, on the great importance of what is termed lateral or oblique illumination in detecting diseases of the anterior part of the eye. A good rule to follow in ophthalmoscopic examinations, — one that will save time, facilitate diagnosis, and prevent error, — is to always commence the examination by

LATERAL ILLUMINATION.

Lateral Illumination of the eye is best conducted in a darkened room, also. The patient sits relatively to the light, as in the ophthalmoscopic examination. The convex object glass is to be held between his eye and the light, the patient facing the observer, so that a strong light is thrown obliquely on to the front of the eye illuminating the cornea and anterior chamber. We may in this way detect opacities of the lens, examine with the greatest nicety the surface of the cornea and the texture of the iris. A second convex glass may also be used at the same time to look through as a magnifying power, if desirable.

DIFFICULTIES OF DIAGNOSIS IN DISEASES OF THE EYE, FORMERLY.

Before the discovery of the opthalmoscope, by Helmholz, in 1851, very little, comparatively speaking, was known concerning the internal diseases of the eye, and the little knowledge which we possessed was very inexact. The history and progress of this kind of disease it was of course impossible to determine with any certainty. Diseased eyeballs were rarely dissected after death; and when this was done, it yielded but scanty return for the labor. A comparison of the pathological anatomy in such an instance, with the symptoms observed during life, in an organ of which nothing objective, in regard to its deeper structures, could be previously determined, afforded little satisfaction, and still less serviceable information. We may say, therefore, that previous to the introduction of the opthalmoscope, our entire knowledge, almost, of the diseases of those parts of the eye posterior to the crystalline lens was conjectural. When the cornea and the iris and the lens presented no appearances of lesion, and yet the patient's visual power was impaired, we were disposed, and it might be said perhaps that we were compelled, *nolens volens*, to attribute the visual disturbance to some affection of the optic nerve. In the words of another, when neither the patient nor the doctor could see any thing, it was amaurosis! * Now we are enabled to determine not only the existence of an amaurosis, but what is sometimes of still greater practical importance, to determine what is not an amaurosis. All the less important disorders in the fundus of the globe are exposed to our careful inspection, and we are enabled to treat them understandingly.

---

* Amaurosis sei jener Zustand wo der Kranke nichts sieht und auch der Arzt nichts. — *Walther.*

IMPORTANCE OF THE OPHTHALMOSCOPE TO THE GENERAL PRACTITIONER.

It is within a short time only that, in the treatment of general nervous disorders, the attention of the profession has been called to the importance of knowing the exact condition of what has been fitly termed the outpost of the central nervous system, — the nervous structure of the posterior portion of the eye, the condition of which gives, to a great extent, a faithful picture of the condition of the brain itself. The ophthalmoscope is, therefore, destined in the future to be of great service to physicians in the treatment of a large class of diseases of the brain and nervous system. Among disorders of this kind which the general practitioner is called upon to treat, and in which the ophthalmoscope has already proved serviceable as an aid to diagnosis, to their pathology, and to a more complete understanding of their history, are the following: meningitis, encephalitis, hydrocephalus, cerebral hemorrhage, tumors, epilepsy, insanity, locomotor ataxy, nervous fevers, and myelitis. These are all known to be accompanied by changes in the appearance of the optic nerve and retina, which can be seen and recognized through the ophthalmoscope.

In the optic nerve disc, for instance, we may see congestion and effusion, inflammation of substance and sheath, anæmia, and atrophy. An optic neuritis is connected with meningitis of the base of the brain, with a tumor, with large hemorrhage. An atrophy of the nerve, which may be recognized as either progressive or stationary, is accompanied by disease of the brain, cerebellum, or spinal cord. In lead poisoning, a German physician has noticed a change of color and transparency in the optic nerve disc. In the retina, we detect inflammations, fatty or fibrous exudations, and hemorrhages; in the choroid, loss or disturbance of pigment, hemorrhages, and effusions; and in the blood-vessels of the fundus generally are observed diminution in size, dilatation, obliteration, tortuosities, pulsations, varicosities, blood stases, displacement, effusion, and rupture. In albuminuria or Bright's disease, one may see extravasations along the course of the retinal vessels, which later become effusions, forming white patches. Finally, there is degeneration of the substance of the retina, and defective nutrition of the optic nerve. In syphilis, we find a retino-choroiditis, with white, red, and brown patches.

In meningitis, Bouchut* has observed, in fifty-nine cases, obvious changes in the eye of all but two. In the first stage, there is dilatation of the veins of the

* Medico-Chir. Review, January, 1868

retina, peri-papillary congestion, and often effusion. In the second stage, there are "tortuous veins, stasis, thrombosis, and even rupture of the vessels." Sometimes the first noticeable symptom of the disease is found in the eye. To be able to diagnose an obscure case of meningitis from a nervous fever, in an early stage of the disease, is of great practical importance. In hydrocephalus, the same observer has noticed numerous and enlarged retinal vessels, and a prominent and suffused optic disc. He remarks that the ophthalmoscope is of the greatest service in diagnosing this affection; and that without its aid, diagnosis of chronic cases may sometimes be impossible.

Chronic headache, especially when the location of the pain is unusual or seems permanently fixed, and when accompanied by vomiting, should be regarded with suspicion, and every means taken to determine the state of the brain. Severe headaches and bilious vomiting, have been known to herald final disease of the brain, and amaurosis. The ophthalmoscope will often be of value in enabling the practitioner to determine the significance of these symptoms, whether they are to be regarded as of cerebral or of gastric origin, — a most important question and often difficult to decide.

In insanity, the ophthalmoscope bids fair to be

come an important agent in determining its course. Of a large number of patients already submitted to examination, two-thirds have been found to present affections of the optic nerve. Dr. Allbutt, of the Leeds Infirmary, found that in fifty-three cases of that kind of insanity known as general paralysis, forty-one had disease of the optic nerve. The affection begins as a pink suffusion of the disc, and ends in white atrophy. It resembles in appearance the "red and white" softening of the brain. Of fifty-one cases of mania, more than half showed symptoms of disease of the optic nerve, — a stasis followed by consecutive atrophy, or white, or mixed atrophy. After a paroxysm, there is a paralysis of the blood-vessels, and about the disc, causing hyperæmia. In dementia and in idiocy more than half; and in insanity, from epilepsy, a large number of cases showed disease of the optic nerve or retina.

The eye has also been observed after the administration of chloroform, when temporary congestion of the vessels of the retina and capillary effusion, rendering the optic disc indistinct, were found. After large doses of opium and belladonna, nearly the same effects were observed. Prof. Graefe has published some interesting ophthalmoscopic observations upon the retina of cholera patients. He found invariably stagnation of blood in the branches of the arteria centralis retinæ, and the retinal veins were unusually dark. The optic disc was of pale lilac color, faded towards its centre. Of course, investigations of this nature are of little consequence, as showing simply the state of the eye, regarded by itself as an organ apart from the brain. In the treatment of a case of cholera, or even in the diagnosis of a case of cholera, the ophthalmoscopic appearance of the eye is a matter of the least possible import; but when we regard the vascular and nervous structure of the fundus of the eye as a picture in miniature of the condition of the brain itself, the importance of researches of this kind can hardly be overstated.

Thus investigations in regard to the diseases involving the brain and nervous system are being pushed rapidly forward, through ocular examination of the nervous and vascular tissues of the eye with the ophthalmoscope. For the first time we *see* a diseased nerve, and measure with our eye the progress of the affection. It has been remarked with truth that hereafter no record of a nervous affection can be considered complete unless it gives a faithful account of the ophthalmoscopic appearance of the retina and optic nerve.

CHAPTER IV.

REFRACTION, ACCOMMODATION, AND THEIR ANOMALIES.

Refraction of the eye, or the refractive power of the eye, is the phrase used to express the power of the cornea and lens to bring rays of light entering the pupil to a focus in the vicinity of the retina.

Accommodation expresses the ability of the eye to increase or lessen its refractive power by means of the ciliary muscle and iris. Thus, in a state of rest, regarding a distant object, the emmetropic (normally refractive) eye needs no exercise of its power of accommodation, because the cornea and lens are precisely convex enough to bring parallel or distant rays of light to a focus on the retina. The latter is situated at a distance of about one inch behind the cornea, and the refractive power of the eye at rest is about equivalent to a convex glass of one-inch focus. But if we regard an object near the eye, the rays fall no longer parallel upon the cornea, but divergently, and of course a greater focussing power is needed to bring them to a point at the proper distance behind the lens. A refractive power, the equivalent of a one-inch convex glass, is insufficient, and the exercise of the power of accommodation becomes necessary.

HOW ACCOMMODATION OF THE EYE IS EFFECTED.

The accommodation is brought about by the action of the ciliary muscle upon the crystalline lens, the surface of which is rendered more convex anteriorally and posteriorally, giving it in consequence a higher refractive power. The anterior surface of the lens is also pushed slightly forward. Associated with this, there are also the movements of the iris, the pupil being diminished in size and moved forward, while the periphery of the iris is drawn slightly backward, and in binocular vision the action of the recti interni to produce the necessary convergence of the optic axes.

DISTINCTION BETWEEN REFRACTION AND ACCOMMODATION.

It is to be remarked that the power of accommodation in the eye may be entirely suspended (as for instance by the instillation of a strong solution of atropine), and still the refraction remain sufficient for distant vision. In presbyopia, the accommodation is much lessened in power, so that the near point for fine print may be as far as fifteen inches or further from the eye, while the emmetropic eye is able to see the same print distinctly at three inches. The former, like the latter, has perfect refractive power for distance. In myopia, the antero-posterior diameter of the eyeball being lengthened, the refractive power is too great for distant objects, — the power of accommodation may be unimpaired. In the hypermetropic eye the same diameter is too short; there is a lack of refractive power, — the rays of light reaching the retina before being focussed, — while the accommodative power may be good.

REFRACTION AND ITS ANOMALIES.

Considering rays of light from distant objects as parallel rays, we may say, in general terms, that in the

Emmetropic eye, parallel rays are brought to a focus *upon* the retina.
Myopic eye, " " " " " " " *before* " "
Hypermetropic eye, " " " " " " " *behind* " "
Astigmatic eye, " " " irregularly focussed.

MYOPIA (NEAR-SIGHTEDNESS).

The optical defect of the myopic eye is exactly the reverse of that of the hypermetropic; that is, its refractive power being in excess, parallel rays of light are brought to a focus before reaching the retina. It was supposed formerly that in myopia the cornea was too convex and prominent, but exact measurements have proved the cornea to be less rather than more convex, and although the antero-posterior diameter is lengthened, the bulging of the globe is wholly posterior, at the entrance of the optic nerve. The retina is thus pushed too far back from the cornea and lens. This elongation of the posterior pole of the eyeball can be seen by requesting the patient to look as far inward as possible; we then notice also that the space in the orbit between the outer canthus and the globe, observable in the emmetropic (normally refractive), and especially in the hypermetropic eye, is completely filled up by the distended globe. When the affection is of a high grade, a dazzling sensation is present in a bright light, and there is also more or less amblyopia; the cause of these symptoms will become apparent when we come to notice the condition of the interior of the eye. Myopia is often congenital, and sometimes hereditary, but it is in all probability still oftener acquired. Possibly a predisposition to elongation of the globe, or some malformation of the ball must be present to favor the development of the affection in young persons, but it is nevertheless a fact that certain circumstances produce the disease in apparently well eyes. I speak of it as a disease, and it will be seen presently that a myopic eye is a diseased eye. I have known several students at different times in Vienna, who informed me that when quite young they saw as far as their fellows, but that after commencing their studies, and pursuing them late at night in their homes among the mountains, with no light but that of a miserable tallow candle, and sometimes even less than that, — a shred of cotton in a cup of oil, a light so dim and flickering that the book must approach within a few inches of the eye, or the head be bent over so as nearly to touch the paper when writing, — after studying in this way for a few years they became myopic. We know that myopia is more common among the educated than the illiterate. Soldiers and sailors almost never acquire it, while in schools and colleges it is very common. At one of the colleges at Oxford, 32 in 127 students were myopic. We have even more conclusive proof than this, of the probability that myopia is acquired, in a recent observation of the indefatigable Dr. Hermann Cohn. He found that of 132 compositors, 51.5 per cent were myopic; of these 68 myopes, so large a number as 51 had in early life normal eyes, with unimpaired vision for distance.

Dr. Cohn's researches among school children, if they do not prove the development of myopia in emmetropic eyes, show a fearful controlling influence of certain circumstances in its progress. Of 10,060 school children examined, 1004 were near-sighted: the percentage of myopes increasing from the elementary school upwards, according to the increase of demand for study. For instance, in five village schools the myopia was about $\frac{1}{24}$: that is, the concave glasses required to render vision acute for distance were on the average of about 24-inch focus.

In 22 Elementary schools the myopia averaged about				$\frac{1}{22}$
In 2 Gymnasiums	„	„	„	$\frac{1}{18}$
In 2 Prima (highest school)	„	„	„	$\frac{1}{17}$
In the University (Breslau)	„	„	„	$\frac{1}{14}$

Of the 410 students in the University examined without selection, nearly two-thirds were found near-sighted. Such statistics show but too plainly the progressive nature of the affection. Another remarkable fact brought to light by these researches is that of the apparent infrequency, comparatively speaking, of a hereditary cause; of all these 10,060 children, only 28 had near-sighted father or mother.

Diagnosis.—The diagnosis of myopia is not difficult. It must not be taken for granted, however, that because a patient holds his book too near, or because he does not see well at a distance, he is therefore near-sighted. Astigmatism, and especially hypermetropia, may equally produce defective vision, characterized by such symptoms. Still, no opacities of the cornea or lens being present, if the indistinctness of vision increases very rapidly, as large letters are removed from the eye, we may be tolerably certain of myopia. A better test is to hold before the eyes weak concave glasses, say of 30 or 40 inch focus. If the patient sees better, he is in a great majority of instances near-sighted. Occasionally, however, persons of good accommodative power see more distinctly, for the moment, through weak concave glasses, though not myopic, and sometimes when a very high degree of myopia is present weak concaves are of almost imperceptible benefit; therefore, to make our diagnosis certain, it is better to ascertain beforehand about the number of the glass required to correct the myopia. This may be done by finding the farthest point at which the patient can read the finest type, such as "Brilliant," and if this be at a distance of six, eight, or ten inches from the eye, we may place before his eyes concave glasses of a corresponding number; if his far point is eight inches, a concave glass of eight-inch focus will enable him to see well at a distance, and the existence of myopia is demonstrated beyond a doubt. Another ready and convenient proceeding for the diagnosis of either near sight or oversight is mentioned under the head of Hypermetropia at page 57.

Myopia is also readily diagnosed with the ophthalmoscope. For this purpose we use the erect image (simply the mirror, without the convex object glass), and find that we can see the optic nerve disc and retinal vessels, when the pupil is large, distinctly at a short distance from the eye. On moving our head to either side we find the image moves in the opposite direction; we obtain an inverted image of the fundus of the globe exactly the reverse of that obtained in the hypermetropic eye under a similar examination. For detailed examination of the fundus, especially if the pupil be small, the indirect mode of examination with the object glass is better and more convenient. We may then discover in a majority of cases where the myopia is marked, a staphyloma posticum, which is recognized as a brilliant white or yellowish-white crescent around the edge of the optic nerve disc. It is sometimes narrow, distinct, and regular in outline, extending quite around the disc, but oftener seen only on the side of the disc towards the macula lutea. The crescent is also frequently irregular in shape, broadest towards the yellow spot, its edge indistinct and marked here and there at its margin by patches of black pigment. This appearance is noticed chiefly in progressive myopia, and is the result of a *sclerotico-choroiditis posterior*, and as it progresses we notice a hyperæmic condition and gradual enlargement of the crescent, — small white patches appear at the macula lutea, coalesce and form a union with the crescent about the nerve disc. Vision becomes impaired as the region of the macula lutea is invaded. Vitreous opacities are present as a result of the choroiditis. The vision of the patient is troubled by fixed scotoma, or floating films and shreds, and detachment of the retina from the choroid, or even glaucoma may supervene.

Pathology. — The pathological changes in myopia and staphyloma posticum, and an accompanying sclerotico-choroiditis, consist chiefly in an atrophy of the choroid resulting from the inflammation. This occurring principally around the nerve entrance, permitting the white sclerotic to shine through, we have, as a result, the characteristic crescent so often observed with the ophthalmoscope. The irregular deposit of pigment is owing to the same cause as are also the exudations into the vitreous, and the final separation of the retina to a greater or less extent from the choroid. There is also a thinning of the sclerotic coat, in the vicinity of the optic nerve entrance, and particularly at the apex of the staphyloma. With the choroid the retina suffers also, and finally becomes atrophied in the region of the optic nerve and macula lutea.

The characteristic ophthalmoscopic symptoms spoken of may also be observed when no staphyloma or bulging of the globe obtains, being the result simply of a posterior choroiditis or sclerotico-choroiditis. In the greater number of cases of myopia of the medium and severer grades, ranging from $\frac{1}{15}$ or $\frac{1}{12}$ up to $\frac{1}{4}$, an inflammatory condition of the fundus of the globe, with or without the bulging, exists; hence the inference, that *a myopic eye is a diseased eye.* The same cannot, as a rule, be said of the presbyopic, hypermetropic or astigmatic eye. These names convey the idea simply of certain optical defects. The popular notion, therefore, that a near-sighted eye is *par excellence* a strong eye, is erroneous. No doubt this error arises from the fact so generally noticeable that myopes see fine objects near the eye in a very dim light, and that presbyopia occurs rather later in life. It is true also that the myope, if his eye continue tolerably healthy until advanced in life, finds distant vision somewhat improved. This is due to a diminution in the size of the pupil, and a senile change in the convexity of the lens.

Treatment. — For the purpose of treatment, it is convenient to divide myopia into the *stationary* and *progressive.* Strictly speaking, however, stationary myopia is very rare. It may occur exceptionally, and undoubtedly occurs oftenest in the least severe cases, such as those of from $\frac{1}{20}$ to $\frac{1}{60}$, and in persons above the age of twenty-five or thirty. Wecker*

---

* Maladies des Yeux. Par L. Wecker. Paris, 1867. Tome second, p. 707.

has examined and recorded carefully the status of 2500 cases of myopia. Many of these have been re-examined after the lapse of months or years, and he is led to conclude, from results thus obtained, that myopia is almost invariably more or less progressive. If, however, we are satisfied that in a given case it is non-progressive, we have only to prescribe for our patient the proper concave spectacles, and we have afforded him all the necessary treatment.

In youth, however, almost all myopia *is* progressive, and *progressive myopia threatens blindness.* It does not always lead to blindness by any means, but it *may* lead to it. Staphyloma posticum being present, there is no particular limit to the bulging of the sclerotic, and the consequent or accompanying inflammation and degeneration resulting. The progress of the disease may be exceedingly slow, but at middle age or before, a myopia with staphyloma posticum sometimes reaches a fatal termination, so far as sight is concerned.

Suppose this fatal termination escaped, amblyopia is the invariable accompaniment of a high degree of myopia. A myopic eye of $\frac{1}{6}$, $\frac{1}{5}$, $\frac{1}{4}$, or $\frac{1}{3}$, armed with the proper glass, possesses an acuteness of vision, calling normal vision = 1, frequently of only $\frac{1}{3}$, $\frac{1}{4}$, or $\frac{1}{5}$ after middle life. There is a feeling of fulness and tension of the globe, and, owing to its increased length, the lateral movements of the ball are somewhat limited. There is frequently pain in and around the globe, which is rapidly increased by use of the eyes for reading, especially by artificial light, and muscular asthenopia is often present. If there is much atrophy of the choroid and loss of pigment, the dazzling in a bright light becomes annoying. In cases like these, where the amblyopia is considerable, no glasses can safely be permitted the patient for near objects, for concave lenses diminishing the size of the object, the print for instance, is brought very near the eye. This is injurious, as it overtaxes the accommodative power, requires extreme convergence of the visual axes, thereby causing pressure of the external muscles upon the eyeball, tending to enlarge the posterior staphyloma. It is especially this strong convergence of the visual axes which favors the progress of high degrees of myopia, for those who accommodate for near and fine objects, using but one eye for the purpose, such as watch-makers, are comparatively exempt from the affection. Strong convergence of the eyes for near objects is then to be particularly avoided.

When the eye is irritable, the conjunctiva injected, the ophthalmoscope showing a hyperæmic condition of the nerve disc with or without staphyloma posticum and the patient complains of pain around and sometimes in the eye, with feeling of tension and heaviness in the eyeball, the prescription of glasses should be temporarily delayed until, by complete rest of the eyes and proper remedial measures, the irritable state of the eye is removed. Gentle use of the eye douche will be found grateful, also a lotion composed of a drachm of sp. ether nit. to six or eight ounces of pure water, to which may be added a few drops of aromatic vinegar, the wash to be sponged over the closed lids and about the eye several times a day and allowed to evaporate. At other times a weak collyrium to be dropped into the eye will do better. Such collyria may be made of ten or fifteen grs. of borax, two or three grs. of alum, a grain of sulph. of zinc, each to one or two ounces of water. Occasionally when the congestion has been markedly venous I have applied a lotion of ten to twenty drops of hamamelis to a cup of water, at the same time administering ham. internally.* Frequently, however, a wash of simple tepid milk and water is best, the slightest irritant causing too great reaction. When the congestion and heat are considerable, I give acon. Far more frequently, however, this is not demanded, and macrot., spig., and bell. are more serviceable.

Cactus is admirable also, especially if the ophthal-

---

* *Vide* Hyperæmia of the Conjunctiva.

moscope show a hyperæmia of the optic nerve and retina. Many other and perhaps an entirely different class of remedies may be indicated from other general disturbance in the patient's health, the general health of the patient being of paramount importance in nearly all cases of disease of the eye. The treatment of choroiditis is spoken of elsewhere.

Spectacles. — Generally speaking, no preliminary treatment is called for, and our first step is to select the appropriate spectacles. When the irritability of the eye is not too great, spectacles, instead of retarding, are a potent auxiliary in hastening a cure. They are to be selected with the greatest care. If too weak, they are comparatively useless; if too strong, a positive injury. The degree of myopia is determined by the negative focus of the glass which neutralizes it. If a patient reads No. 1 of the test type at six or eight inches, his myopia is $\frac{1}{6}$ or $\frac{1}{8}$. A concave glass of six or eight inches focus should, theoretically speaking, enable him to read No. 20 at twenty feet, and to see well at a distance. Practically, however, we find it necessary to prescribe concave spectacles rather weaker than this. If the myopia is $\frac{1}{8}$, vision will be most perfect through glasses of $\frac{1}{9}$ or $\frac{1}{10}$, which of the two numbers will prove best is to be determined by trial. The reason of this non-correspondence of the number of glass to the degree of myopia is this: the patient's far point being eight inches, the visual axes were converged for this distance, and with convergence of the eyes is associated accommodation or an increased convexity of the crystalline lens; in looking at a distance through the prescribed glasses, the visual axes are of course parallel, and there being no accommodative power (increased convexity of the crystalline lens) to overcome, the glasses must be proportionally weaker. The proper glass to enable him to read music or small print at twenty-four inches would be of about twelve-inch focus. The formula is this: $-\frac{1}{8}+\frac{1}{24}=-\frac{1}{12}$. The patient's power of accommodation will influence greatly the choice of spectacles. When little or no accommodative power exists, as is often the case in a high grade of myopia, spectacles may be given which completely neutralize the myopia and entirely supplant any little accommodative power present. When only a tolerable power of accommodation is found, it is advisable to prescribe glasses which partially supplant it. Thus if our patient has a myopia of $\frac{1}{8}$, and finds glasses of $\frac{1}{9}$ best, if his power of accommodation be $\frac{1}{12}$, he will, through these glasses, be obliged to use his whole power of accommodation for reading at a distance of twelve inches. This is not safe, lest symptoms of fatigue supervene, his eye become irritable and his myopia be increased.

He should, therefore, be provided with weaker spectacles for reading; concave glasses for instance of sixteen or eighteen inch focus, by diminishing but little the convexity of his crystalline lens enable him to see easily at ten or twelve inches, and tolerably at a short distance beyond. He should therefore, like the myope without accommodation, provide himself with two pairs of glasses, one for reading and one for distance. If *perfect* accommodation is present, as is sometimes the case in the slighter forms of myopia in young persons, a single pair of glasses which neutralize the near-sightedness may be worn for both far and near vision. Generally speaking, though, it is best to prescribe concave spectacles for near objects which only *partially* neutralize the myopia, and enable him to read comfortably at fourteen or sixteen inches. Rules are often however of little practical service. The myopia must be neutralized by suitable glasses whether their strength correspond or not to the apparent degree of near sight. Frequently very strong glasses will be necessary for distant vision, and the patient will find it convenient to carry eye-glasses to use temporarily before his spectacles. These eye-glasses must, of course, be concave and of just the power to supplement the spectacles sufficiently to neutralize the myopia for distant vision. When the myopia is slighter than $\frac{1}{14}$ or $\frac{1}{18}$, fine print being read easily at fourteen inches, spectacles need not be prescribed, but simply the proper eye-glasses for distant vision.

Too great care cannot be exercised in the choice of spectacles in progressive near sight, nor can spectacles be provided too early for children after their education has commenced. The chief danger in the selection of spectacles is that of getting them too strong * and so overtaxing the eyes for near objects. Wecker believes the great prevalence of myopia in Germany to be due partly to wearing too strong glasses. I believe it due principally to the peculiar text in which their books are mostly printed. It requires too sharp vision and too close attention to distinguish the letters. I can never read it long by artificial light without causing asthenopic symptoms, and I have no doubt that the change to the Roman letter, now going on in Germany, will eventually prove of great advantage to its students.

Spectacles, therefore, should not be bought at random of opticians or itinerant venders, but should be prescribed by a competent physician or oculist. The result of random spectacle-buying is seen in Dr. Cohn's report. Of 1004 near-sighted children, only

* Wecker's rule is very good in doubtful cases: "Eviter de donner dans l'hypermétropie des verres trop faibles, et d'en prescrire de trops forts dans la myopie."

107 wore glasses at all. Of this number, 11 only wore glasses which were not injurious to the eye! Of these children 99 had selected their own glasses. Only 8 had glasses selected by a physician or oculist. It is well to determine the amount of myopia for each eye separately, as the refractive power of the two eyes sometimes differs. The glasses should be selected for the least myopic eye as a rule. When one eye is myopic and the other hypermetropic, the most serviceable eye should alone be provided for. If we prescribe a concave for one and a convex glass for the other, the former diminishing and the latter magnifying objects, it will be difficult to fuse the different sized images on the retina. Actual trial, however, is the best method of determining these matters. The best rules have their exceptions. I have a patient whose right eye is myopic and astigmatic, and whose left eye is hypermetropic. For the first he wears an 18-inch concave cylindrical, and for the second a 16-inch convex spherical glass, and with these reads more comfortably with both eyes than with either eye alone.

The phosphenes, spectra, flashes of colored light, and like phenomena, arise from over-sensibility of the retina, and generally disappear under treatment of the irritable condition of the eye. If they do not, like muscæ volitantes and scotoma, they will be rendered less apparent and troublesome by the use of blue glasses.

After prescribing with the greatest care the proper glasses, it is necessary in progressive myopia to enforce the strictest hygienic measures. Our patient should not work continuously at near objects, but should rest a short time at intervals of a quarter or half hour, and always whenever the eyes feel in the least fatigued. He should never work or read with the head bent forward, as this promotes intraocular congestion, choroiditis and increase of staphyloma posticum. The light should fall upon his work from behind, so that the eye may be protected from glare. Children's school desks should, therefore, be made sufficiently high and sufficiently sloping, and be placed, as regards light, to fulfil these conditions. It is almost needless to add that in the modern school-room this is not the case. I remember a humble school-house in the country, where, thirty years or more ago, these conditions *were* fulfilled. The desks were high and very sloping, and running along the sides and across the ends of the room, were all excellently lighted. I never saw a near-sighted boy in those days. Dr. Cohn found all the school furniture badly constructed. Low desks and bad light frequently compelled the scholars to bend over so as to bring the head within three or four inches of the book. It is the duty of physicians everywhere to enlighten parents and teachers in regard to this fatal defect in school-room furniture.

In very high degrees of myopia, such as $\frac{1}{4}$, $\frac{1}{3}$, or $\frac{1}{2}$, even if no amblyopia be present, we cannot expect the patient to read large print through his glasses at a point as distant as a normal eye would do it. The powerful concave glasses diminish the size of the image too much. Very strong concaves are also inconvenient to the wearer, by compelling him to move his head always in looking to the right or left. His glasses are so deeply hollowed that he must always look through their centre, or they produce the effect of prisms or decentred glasses. If the glasses produce dazzling, they may be slightly tinted with blue.

MUSCULAR ASTHENOPIA,

Or insufficiency of the recti interni, is not unfrequent in the severer grades of myopia. It gives rise to confusion of sight and fatigue of the eye, similar to that described under the head of Accommodative Asthenopia. It is caused by overtaxing the internal recti in converging the eyes so as to bring both optic axes to bear at once on near objects. Greater convergence being necessary for myopes, this class suffer oftenest from this affection. It may occur temporarily after exhaustive diseases, such as diphtheria and various kinds of fevers.

DIAGNOSIS.

Let the patient fix his eyes on our finger, and as we approach it to within five or six inches of his eyes, the weaker internus will suddenly relax, and one eye will roll outwards. We may measure the weakness of the muscle by means of prisms. A normal rectus internus will successfully resist the tendency to the production of diplopia of a prism of from 20° to 30°, its base outward. If, therefore, we find double images caused by a prism of 6° or 8°, we may judge as to the degree of weakness of the internal muscles. The action of prisms is further explained under Paralysis of the Ocular Muscles.

TREATMENT.

The treatment will consist, generally, in presenting the proper concave glasses so as to enable the patient to read at a distance of twelve or fifteen inches, in order to avoid great and prolonged convergence of the visual axes. If this does not cure, the general muscular system of the patient being in good condition, we may divide the recti externi, one at a sitting, or only one externus, if this is sufficient to admit of the necessary convergence of the eyes for near vision. The operation is described under the head of Strabismus. Muscular asthenopia, due to general debility after serious illness or other causes, will be cured by such internal treatment and hygienic measures as are necessary for the restoration of the usual health and muscular energy. See Hyperæmia of the Conjunctiva.

HYPERMETROPIA AND ASTHENOPIA (ACCOMMODATIVE).

HYPERMETROPIA,

As we have already seen, is that condition of the eye in which its antero-posterior diameter is too short in comparison with the refractive power (convexity) of the crystalline lens and cornea. The rays of light consequently reach the retina before they are brought to a focus, forming circles of diffusion, and vision is indistinct. A convex glass, or spectacles, by supplementing the refractive power of the natural lens, enables the patient to focus the rays of light upon the retina, precisely as in presbyopia. In presbyopia, however, rays of light from a distance — that is, what are termed parallel rays — are brought to a focus on the retina without the use of accommodating power; while, in hypermetropia, the exercise of this power is always necessary, even for distant vision: and, in the higher grades of the affection, convex glasses are also necessary for all distances. A hypermetropic eye is generally smaller in all its dimensions than the emmetropic or normally refractive, and is probably of congenital and hereditary source.

Hypermetropia is divided by Donders into *facultative*, *relative* and *absolute*.

Facultative is the slightest form, where the patient accommodates readily for all distances; presbyopia occurs rather early, and then asthenopic symptoms are apt to occur; while, in

Relative hypermetropia, although the patient can accommodate so as to see well at all distances, yet this is only accomplished through great efforts of accommodation, and by converging the optic axes too much at the same time. Such persons are almost certain to become asthenopic.

Absolute hypermetropia is a condition of the eye in which the patient sees distinctly only by the aid of convex glasses. Without spectacles no effort of accommodation, however great, will suffice to prevent rays of light reaching the retina before being brought to a focus.

DIAGNOSIS.

Let the patient look at No. 20 of the test type at twenty feet, and if his vision is improved by looking through convex glasses of 30, 40, or 50 inch focus he is hypermetropic. These glasses would not render the vision of an emmetropic eye more acute. But it may happen that, although slightly hypermetropic, he does not see as well through the convex glasses, or he may even see as well, through concave glasses of thirty or forty inch negative focus, as in myopia. He is not myopic, however; but in looking through the concave glasses he involuntarily exerts all his power of accommodation; and when this power is considerable he overcomes, for the time being, his own as well as the additional hypermetropia caused by the concave glasses. Ordinarily, however, we find that a weak convex glass improves vision; if it does not, we may try the effect of paralyzing the accommodation by the instillation of atropine. We can then determine the whole extent of the hypermetropia, both latent and manifest. If after an hour or two we try our convex glasses again, we may find that whereas, previously he could only see well through convex thirty, he now sees best through convex twelve or fifteen. His manifest hypermetropia was only one-thirtieth; but his latent, being added, gives him really a hypermetropia of one-twelfth or one-fifteenth. It is advisable, however, to avoid the use of atropine on account of the inconvenience which a solution sufficiently strong to paralyze the accommodation causes the patient in the disturbance of vision for several days, and to this end the following method will be serviceable.

It will be remembered that the retina is so near the lens that rays of light reach the former before being focussed; the eye is for ever accommodated for a point beyond the object. It is *over*-sighted. Now, if we place before an emmetropic eye a convex glass of eight-inch focus, it will be able to read No. 1 test type at a distance of eight inches, for the rays of light coming to the eye through this lens are rendered parallel, just as they would be if they came from a distance or the *far* point of the eye. If we find, however, on applying this test, that the type can be distinctly seen through our No. 8 convex glass no nearer than at nine, ten, or eleven inches, we are sure that we have an oversighted or hypermetropic eye. This test also proves an eye to be myopic if it sees the type best at a distance *less* than eight inches from the eye. Another, and very simple test, for anomalous refraction, without the aid of glasses, is mentioned under Amblyopia.

We may diagnose the affection also by means of the ophthalmoscope, using the direct image. With this we see the details of the fundus at a little distance, as in myopia, only in this instance we get our image uninverted. A movement to the right or left will produce a similar movement in the image, and not the reverse as in myopia. Approaching nearer, we find the field of vision unusually large, and the optic disc apparently small, but very distinct, just the reverse of what we notice in myopia. If we use the indirect mode of examination with the object glass, we find the disc to appear larger than usual in other refractive states of the eye.

In the higher grades of hypermetropia we often find, especially in young children, a convergent strabismus. The accommodative effort of the eye is always accompanied by a slight convergence of the optic axes. These consentaneous movements in the normal eye are necessary for acute visual power in regarding near objects. For distance, no accommodation being necessary, no convergence takes place. With the relative or absolute hypermetropic eye all this is different. It is obliged to accommodate for all distances, and with accommodation comes convergence, and in course of time a periodic strabismus becomes fixed and permanent.

Spectacles *for distance* should not be prescribed for hypermetropia, if the patient can see well and without fatigue, as, after being used for distant vision, they become indispensable for all time; but, for near vision, they should be ordered the moment asthenopic symptoms appear. In higher grades of the affection, where vision for all distances is imperfect, glasses which correct the *manifest* hypermetropia should first be worn; and later, when the eyes become accustomed to these, stronger ones should be prescribed, if necessary, so as to correct more or less of the *latent* defect also.

ASTHENOPIA

May be defined as a condition of the eye in which it cannot be used continuously for near vision, even in the best light, without pain and confusion of sight, although for the first moment the patient sees with ease and distinctness. The eyes are sound in appearance, in movement, in visual form, in convergence of visual axes, but they rebel against all use, however moderate. After the least service upon near objects, they feel fatigued, full, hot, and sometimes become quite painful; the pain extending to the head, or following the branches of the fifth nerve.

It is not unusual for asthenopic eyes to show a slight hyperæmia of the conjunctiva, and sometimes we notice an enlarged and rather sluggish pupil. The dilated pupil is not due to any local disease, but to reflex disturbance of the ciliary nerves from irritation of the sympathetic. In these cases we find spinal irritation or disturbance of the uterine or digestive functions. The dilatation of the pupil is, when it exists, an additional hindrance to distinct vision for near objects, by admitting too much light and too many lateral rays, and by increasing the circles of diffusion. As the rays reach the retina before being focussed the object is not pictured upon the retina at a single point, but by a number of conical pencils of rays in the form of circles which overlapping each other, render the image blurred. The ophthalmoscopic signs are usually negative. The media are clear, and there are no striking anomalies of refraction. Sometimes, however, there is to be observed a hyperæmic condition of the optic nerve disc, and retina similar to the hyperæmic state of the conjunctiva. In rare instances, the optic nerve itself appears to be the principal seat of the pain. I can recall instances where the least exercise of the eye produced deep-seated pain of the globe. *The cause of this affection* is the characteristic formation of the eye which renders it hypermetropic.

Formerly, asthenopia was looked upon as a grave affection, and as a probable precursor of amaurosis, or some other disease fatal to sight. More recently, it has been regarded as a symptom of general debility, arising from exanthematous or febrile affections, from overwork, mental troubles, dissipations, abuse of the eyes, and like causes. All these, however, only express the occasional, or exciting, cause. The primary cause is to be sought in a more or less faulty state of the refractive power of the eye, and the faulty refraction is a hypermetropia. We can now explain very readily the mystery of some eyes giving out upon the least abuse or overwork, or deterioration of the general health; while others bear any amount of fine work night or day, and, in failure of the general health, are the last to be affected. The first are hypermetropic, and have always required extra exertion of the ciliary muscle in accommodating for near vision; while the second are emmetropic, or as nearly this as possible, and, the apparatus of accommodation having necessarily been used with moderation, its integrity is preserved. Some hypermetropic eyes escape asthenopia for a longer time also, on account of having been originally endowed with a wider power of accommodation. A youthful normal eye is sometimes able to read the finest type, No. 1, from three up to eighteen inches, while another may be able to read it only from four up to twelve inches: the first showing an accommodative power of considerably greater range than the second. Moreover, according to Graefe, there is considerable difference exhibited by different individuals in the impunity with which they may exert a great part of the accommodative power at their disposal. Some persons, for instance, are unable to use one-half of this power for any length of time without injury, while others use more than three-quarters without fatigue. In the first, there appears to be a lack of energy in the ciliary muscle: while, in the second, it is unusually vigorous. Hence it may follow that the more or less perfect optical construction shall in some instances give but an imperfect indication of the serviceableness of an eye for fine work. This, however, is certain, that the greatest amount of muscular energy, and the widest range of accommodation, cannot prevent an excessively hypermetropic eye from becoming asthenopic.

TREATMENT OF ACCOMMODATIVE ASTHENOPIA AND HYPERMETROPIA.

The first and most important indication in the treatment of asthenopia is to relieve the painful and overworked ciliary muscle by supplementing the refractive power of the crystalline lens with suitable convex glasses. We have by no means finished our treatment, however, when we have prescribed convex spectacles for our patient. We must still keep him under our control, to determine whether the glasses are affording him the requisite relief; whether we have perhaps prescribed a too weak or too strong pair, and whether they are invariably worn for near objects, as directed.

Sometimes, when the affection is of long standing, and the whole eye seems to have been reduced to an extremely irritable and sensitive condition, we may have considerable trouble in finding glasses that can be worn with comfort; and yet, if the eyes are to be used at all, the help of glasses is absolutely required. It may be necessary in those cases to completely paralyze the accommodation for some weeks by the instillation of atropine, simply for the purpose of resting the eye.

For the selection of glasses, I generally determine the amount of manifest hypermetropia, by permitting the patient to look at No. 20 print at a distance of twenty feet, or where an emmetropic eye would see it with distinctness. Then I find the lowest convex glass through which he can read the print, and this determines the degree of manifest hypermetropia. In the great majority of cases of asthenopia, the convex glass will be about thirty-six or forty inches. Having determined this point, I prescribe, if the hypermetropia is thirty-six, a convex glass of thirty-inch focus; if it is fifty, glasses of about forty-inch focus, and so on. Wecker advises that the manifest and about one-fourth of the latent hypermetropia should be corrected by the first glasses presented. I notice, in looking over my records of quite a large number of cases of asthenopia, glasses of thirty-inch focus are prescribed oftener than any other; and the cases occur almost invariably in persons from fifteen to thirty years of age. I find nearly twice as many cases in females as in males; but this is probably not owing to a preponderance of hypermetropia in females, but rather to the fact that their occupation in general, and especially by artificial light in the evening, requires greater exertion of the accommodative power of the eye than that of males. Collegians and accountants, among the latter, are frequent sufferers.

It will often be necessary to change the glasses, after a few weeks, for those of greater refractive power, in order to cure the asthenopia. Sometimes, in asthenopia due to facultative hypermetropia, the glasses, after having served to cure the asthenopic symptoms, may be discarded. The patient should be particularly enjoined to use *invariably* his spectacles for near vision, and, whenever in any occupation his eyes seem fatigued, to rest a few minutes. In looking at distant objects, although he is obliged to accommodate, it is only momentarily as a rule, and need not, if discretion is used, fatigue the eye much. It is also advisable generally, according to my experience, that the patient should use the eyes daily for near objects, always of course with moderation and discretion, rather than persist in resting them wholly.

If the asthenopia is clearly the result of general debility, due to diminished energy of the muscular system generally, and the hypermetropia is very slight, it is possible that the restoration of vigorous health through internal medication, generous as well as prudent dietetic regulations or change of air, may cure the asthenopia without the necessity of a resort to spectacles at all. The hyperæmia of the conjunctiva common in asthenopia is noticed elsewhere. *The irritability of the eye* is best treated, according to my experience by the internal use of macrot., nux v. spig., and gelsem. when the general symptoms of the patient do not forbid their use. When there is irritability of the sympathetic nerve, nervous dyspepsia, irritation of the uterus or kidneys and sensitiveness of the brain and nervous system generally, these remedies are indicated, aside from the symptoms of the eye itself. Want of appetite also is successfully met by macrot., nervous dyspepsia by nux v. and gelsem., and an appearance of congestion of the tunics of the globe as well as of the nerve disc and retina points to spigel., cactus, and bell. Retinal asthenopia is noticed under Amblyopia.

ASTIGMATISM.

This is an anomaly of refraction dependent generally on a lack of symmetry in the different meridians of the cornea. It was noticed by Young in 1793, but first correctly explained by Donders, who published a work on the subject in 1862. Previous to the researches of Donders, there had been recorded less than a dozen cases, for seventy years; since his investigations, cases are recorded daily. Astigmatism is congenital, or may be acquired from wounds or ulceration of the cornea. It is divided into the *regular* and the *irregular*.

REGULAR ASTIGMATISM

Is called *simple* when one meridian of the cornea is emmetropic and the other myopic or hypermetropic. It is *compound* when both meridians are myopic or hypermetropic, but in different degrees, as if, for instance, in the vertical meridian the cornea were sufficiently convex to make a myopia of $\frac{1}{8}$, while in the horizontal line it might be only convex enough for a myopia of $\frac{1}{16}$. In rare instances there is *mixed astigmatism*, one meridian being myopic, the other hypermetropic.

IRREGULAR ASTIGMATISM

Is due to imperfections in the structure of, or to partial dislocation of the lens, or to its partial opacity. It is found also in conical cornea, and results from ulcerations of the cornea, and occasionally from irregularity of its surface after cataract operations.

DIAGNOSIS AND TREATMENT.

To determine whether a patient is astigmatic we have only to place some rather thick vertical and horizontal lines before him at considerable distance, — perhaps thirty feet, and then gradually approach them so as to find if, at any distance, one set of lines appear clear and the other indistinct. If such a point *can be found* he is astigmatic; if not, we are obliged to refer his defective vision to some other cause.

We must bear in mind that no eye is perfectly symmetrical in form, and so we may expect to find that vertical and horizontal lines will not be seen always with equal distinctness: but usually this asymmetry is so slight that no annoyance in vision is occasioned. Astigmatism is to be suspected when the patient finds no glasses (spherical) which satisfactorily improve his sight.

Having determined the existence of astigmatism, if we permit the patient to hold a metallic disc before the eye, in which there is a slit of about a line or rather less in width, and rotate it until it comes opposite the emmetropic meridian of the cornea, so that rays of light are received by the eye through this meridian alone, he will see distinctly, reading No. 20 at twenty feet. This supposes a case of *simple astigmatism*, one meridian of the cornea being normally refractive or emmetropic. To neutralize this astigmatism and render vision acute, we have only to prescribe weak concave or convex cylindrical glasses.

CYLINDRICAL GLASSES

Are segments of a cylinder, whereas ordinary glasses are segments of a sphere. A concave spherical glass, for instance, increases in thickness from the centre in all directions. A concave cylindrical glass, held with its axis in a horizontal direction, is equally thin throughout in its horizontal plane, but in its vertical plane increases in thickness from the centre like a spherical concave. Those rays of light which strike a cylindrical lens at right angles with the plane of its axis are refracted most, and those which strike *in the plane of its axis* are not refracted at all. Cylindrical glasses are, therefore, unlike spherical, to be rotated before the eye until the plane of their highest refraction comes opposite that plane of the cornea which requires it.

In *compound astigmatism* we proceed to determine first how much we can improve vision by the ordinary glasses, convex or concave. Suppose it a case of myopic astigmatism, and we find sight best through a spherical concave glass of $\frac{1}{20}$. We then select a weak concave cylindrical glass, and placing it before the other allow the patient to look through both, rotating the last until its axis is in the right direction. If it proves too weak we try others. We may determine also, in advance, the number of the cylindrical glass required with tolerable exactness by noting the different strength of two glasses, through one of which horizontal lines are best seen, and through the other of which vertical ones are plainest. Take the two letters on the next page made up of horizontal and vertical lines. A. sees N blackest, but with convex No. 15 sees Z blackest. With cylindrical convex No. 15 axis vertical, his astigmatism will be corrected. B. sees Z blackest through No. 60 concave, and N blackest through No. 20 concave. Then * $-\frac{1}{20}-\frac{1}{60}=-\frac{1}{30}$. A cylindrical —30 glass with the axis horizontal would neutralize his astigmatism.

A color test is recommended by Green, of St. Louis. Bright red and blue, or other shades of these colors, rendered brilliant by transmitted light, as when hung at a window, are most practical. The colors are arranged in radiating lines. For the details of the color test and others, consult the proceedings of the American Ophthalogical Society for the year 1869. I have mentioned also a simple test for astigmatism under Amblyopia.

---

* A concave glass is designated by the sign — and a convex by the sign +.

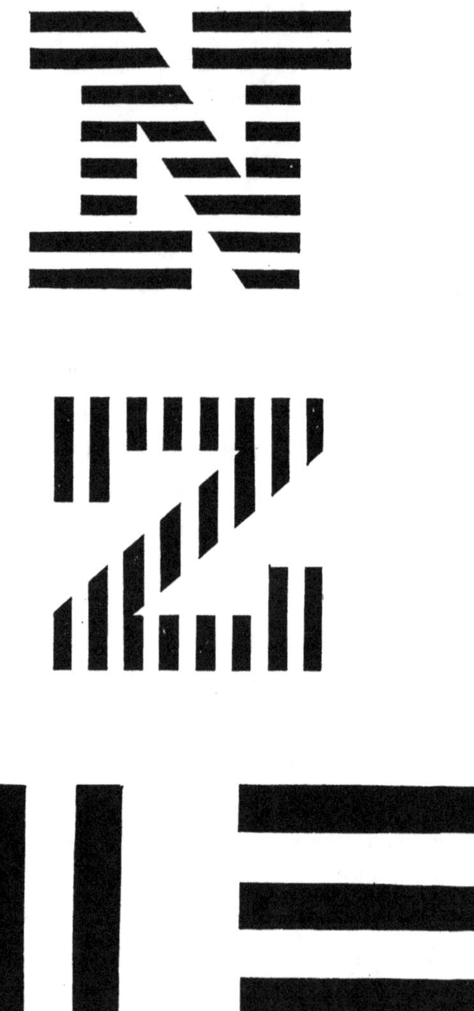

MIXED ASTIGMATISM.

This form requires by-cylindrical glasses for its correction. A plano-cylin. convex glass for the hypermetropic meridian, and a plano-cylin. concave glass for the myopic meridian of the cornea are to be selected and put together, their axes at right angles, then rotated before the eye until their best position is found.

Astigmatism may also be diagnosed with the ophthalmoscope, as mentioned in the chapter preceding, the disc appearing oval instead of circular. Mixed astigmatism has also been diagnosed with the ophthalmoscope by noticing both the erect and inverted image by direct examination of the different meridians of the same eye.

PRESBYOPIA.

Far sight is a symptom of advancing years, and is due to diminished power of accommodation. Distant vision remains good. but no effort of the ciliary muscle is sufficient to render the lens convex enough to bring rays of light from near objects to a focus on the retina. Hence the necessity for convex glasses. It is *not* advisable to postpone the use of glasses as long as possible at the expense of discomfort and fatigue of the eye. The proper glasses for a presbyope are such as will enable him to read No. 1 at ten or twelve inches. It is convenient to have two pairs of spectacles: the stronger one for evening use. *Rapidly increasing presbyopia* is to be viewed with suspicion, as it is often a precursor of glaucoma.

CHAPTER V.

THE CONJUNCTIVA.

HYPERÆMIA OF THE CONJUNCTIVA.

HYPERÆMIA of the conjunctiva is of very common occurrence, and is due to overuse or abuse of the eyes, or to optical defects, as in asthenopia. The appearance of the eye is very similar to that observed in mild conjunctivitis, but there is no discharge from the conjunctiva, and usually very little or no lachrymation, and the smarting, itching, and heaviness of the lids is markedly increased in the evening. Reading by strong artificial light, or by a too weak light, and the very hazardous practice of reading habitually in the horse and steam cars, and that worst and most dangerous of habits for the eyes, that of reading in bed by artificial light — produce constantly this congestion, and if continued, still more serious troubles. This state of the conjunctiva is often a reflex symptom of a similar condition or more serious disease, of the internal structures of the eyes. Use of the eyes for any length of time continuously, increases the unpleasant sensations or the pain and asthenopic symptoms, if such are present.

TREATMENT.

To cure this affection, it is of course necessary to remove its cause. Optical defects must be remedied by appropriate spectacles. Injurious use of the eyes must be given up and overwork proscribed. As palliatives, the use of the eye douche, always with closed lids, is excellent, or bathing in tepid water, or vinegar and water, a few drops of tincture of hamamelis, or tincture of opium, or of hydrastis in a cup of water, or a grain or two of sulphate of zinc, or of acetate of lead — any of these, adhering of course to the one which seems most grateful to the eye, may be used as a fomentation, either warm or cold, to the lids several times a day. If preferred by the patient, these lotions may be used to saturate a bit of lint or linen which may be laid over the lids for a quarter of an hour three or four times a day. The solution need not enter the eye, but will, of course, occasion no pain of consequence in case this should happen. Sometimes, in severe pain, we may prescribe the vapor from ether or chloroform, or from chloroform, to one ounce of which is added a few drops of tincture of iodine, or from bi-sulphuret of carbon, or from spirits of rosemary, to which is added one-eighth its quantity of ether. These should be kept in glass-stoppered, rather wide-mouthed bottles, or cup-mouthed bottles if possible, and when used, the stopper being removed, the bottle is brought near the closed lids, which are subjected to the influence of the vapor a few minutes at a sitting. The palliative and soothing effect of the vapor is sometimes very marked. If the skin is delicate, caution should at first be used both as regards the strength of the application and its repetition. A lotion of bell. ext. twenty grains to four ounces of water as a fomentation will frequently quiet pain but it will enlarge the pupil, which is not always permissible. Irritating collyria, to be dropped into the eye, are not usually serviceable in my experience.

Internally I often administer opium or ham., when prescribing them externally, and also the remedies mentioned under Accommodative Asthenopia. Bell. and conium are also serviceable for the photophobia. In other instances it is necessary to be guided almost wholly by general indications in the selection of remedies, and to look for the improvement in the eyes only through the improving of the impaired health.

CONJUNCTIVITIS.

An inflammation of the conjunctiva is easy to diagnose, and yet a mistake is possible if one is not in the habit of observing accurately the difference in the appearance of a reddened eye in different kinds of inflammation. For instance in the simplest conjunctivitis, in place of the usually invisible vessels of the conjunctiva, we have a network of bright red vessels plainly seen to be superficial and movable by the touch of the finger over the smooth surface of the sclerotica. On the other hand, in a severer, deeper-seated conjunctivitis, like the scrofulous, or lymphatic, and the granular, we may see close parallel lines of immovable subconjunctival vessels running towards the edge of the cornea, forming around its circumference a dull pinkish red zone. In iritis the zone is usually well marked. It is formed by the congestion of the deep-seated vessels of the conjunctiva, and not, as is often supposed, by inflammation of the sclerotic. The congested vessels are on, but not of, the sclerotica. In scleritis, or episcleritis, there is presented still another redness of a violet or purple tinge. It appears nearly always in rather large and tolerably well circumscribed patches, and is sometimes mistaken by the general practitioner for conjunctivitis phlyctenia, although the bright red color and papular appearance of the latter, and the peculiar color of the deep-seated spots of the former, render the differential diagnosis easy.

SIMPLE CONJUNCTIVITIS.

Simple conjunctivitis differs in degree, rather than in form, from the acute catarrhal. It is generally the result of slight injury to the eye, contact of a foreign body, exposure of the eyes to dust, smoke, cold winds or dampness, glare of light, impure air, prolonged exertion in accommodating the eyes for near objects, or from some other local cause. The subjective symptoms are very trivial usually. There may be some itching and sensation of heat in the lids, or a feeling as if there were sand in the eye. We ought to determine by ocular inspection, whenever our patient complains of a sensation as if a foreign body were in the eye, or when a simple conjunctivitis does not yield readily to treatment, whether there may not be some foreign substance lodged beneath the upper lid. The immediate cure of a conjunctivitis after three weeks of ineffectual treatment, by the simple eversion of the upper lid and the removal of a bit of quartz, is mentioned in the chapter on Injuries of the Eye.

CATARRHAL CONJUNCTIVITIS.

The objective symptoms in *catarrhal conjunctivitis* are more marked than in the simple form of the affection. The congestion of the superficial vessels of the conjunctiva is greater, and in elderly people chemosis is usually present. The edges of the lids appear swollen, the palpebral conjunctiva is distended from serous infiltration, particularly at its reflected portion, its papillæ are enlarged, and its surface presents a velvety appearance. There is a secretion of clouded mucus alternating sometimes with a secretion muco-purulent in character. This discharge is often abundant, but rarely as profuse as in purulent conjunctivitis, and is slightly contagious. Probably the contagiousness is in direct ratio to the increased admixture of pus globules in the discharge. A healthy conjunctiva may be successfully inoculated with the secretion of an acute catarrh.

The subjective symptoms are not very characteristic. There is the complaint of not seeing well at a distance, and the common symptom of a feeling at first of dryness, and as if sand or some foreign body were in the eye, and there is a heavy uncomfortable feeling about the lids which leads to a desire to rub them, and frequently a slight burning and smarting sensation is complained of. There is rarely severe pain, nor is the photophobia marked. The above subjective symptoms vanish, to a great extent, as a case becomes chronic. As to the treatment, it should be very simple in acute cases. No doubt acute catarrh of the conjunctiva, under proper hygienic conditions, and under circumstances controlling the causes which have produced it, disappears frequently in the course of a week or two without any treatment whatever. In other cases, however, it will not disappear of itself, and may be sufficiently severe from the commencement to require treatment.

TREATMENT.

In the first or inflammatory stage the cold douche, or cold compresses with the internal administration of acon., will afford great relief, and often effect a cure. No irritating collyria are permissible at this stage. Later, I prefer euph., arsen., nux, hydras, or macrot., and if a considerable muco-purulent discharge continues, then merc., hepar, zinc, and arg-nit. Complications, such as blepharitis, or in rare instances, ulceration of the cornea, or nasal, throat, or bronchial inflammations, may call for other remedies as intercurrents. The exciting cause of the disease, whether exposure, contagion, abuse of the eyes, or the sequence of exanthematous fever will influence, in a degree, the selection of remedies. Simple collyria, such as a solution of five to ten grains of borax, two grains of alum, or one grain of sul. of zinc, one grain of nitrate of silver, each to the ounce of water, will often be found serviceable. I am in the habit of administering the zinc or nit. arg. internally, when prescribing it as a collyrium. If the affection prove very obstinate, and the discharge assume a puriform character, the case should be treated as directed under Purulent Conjunctivitis. A solution of nitrate of silver, of five grains to the ounce of water, may be used, but not as a collyrium. The lids, upper and lower, should be everted, and held in this position with the left hand; the patient should close the eye gently, this will bring the everted lids together and prevent contact with the cornea. The conjunctiva thus exposed is painted by means of a camel's hair pencil with this solution, which after a second or two is immediately washed off with tepid water from another pencil. If the pain is afterwards severe, it will be relieved by bathing the eyes in cold water, by cold compresses, and frequently through simple contact of the eyes with the cool out-door air. Often a few applications like this at infrequent intervals, cures the patient.

The object of the application is to create a slight inflammatory condition *similar to the conjunctivitis;* having occasioned this, the operation should not be repeated until the artificial exacerbation has fully subsided. Probably a repetition two or three times a week will be sufficient.

If active inflammatory symptoms are present, or such as are evinced by a very bright red, congested, and swollen conjunctiva, when the sub-conjunctival vessels are visibly involved, and when the ciliary nervous system is sensitive, as shown by pain and photophobia, irritating applications should never be made. In all cases where irritating collyria are used it is advisable not to push their employment too continuously, but rather alternate them from time to time for a few days with the use of the cold compress. It is always advisable to see that a collyrium which the patient takes home be not too strong. It is necessary also, to remember that in a conjunctivitis occurring in two individuals of different nervous organization, where in each case it seems to be of the same nature and to require the same remedy, one may use a wash with great benefit which the other may be quite unable to bear. Whenever, therefore, there is the least doubt about the strength of the solution it is advisable to instruct the patient that if the pain after its use continues beyond a minute, it is too strong, and it should be diluted with an equal quantity of water. It is safer, also, to direct that the collyrium be used not oftener than twice a day. It has often been my experience when called in consultation with physicians of our school, to find that in conjunctivitis complicated and uncomplicated, collyria when used at all have been frequently too strong, applied too often, and to eyes already too sensitive and irritable.

We should bear in mind the contagiousness of some catarrhs of the conjunctiva. The patient should be warned of this danger, so that he may not propagate the disease. Frequently the affection assumes an epidemic character, attacking whole families and neighborhoods. In the chronic form of this affection the results of topical application to the lids will not prove as satisfactory as in the acute. Improvements will be followed by relapses, and with all the help which homœopathic medication affords, many cases will prove extremely tedious in treatment. If however the affection seems to be purely local and confined to the eyes, our prognosis will be more favorable than when it is merely a part of a catarrhal affection of the air-passages generally or of the lachrymal duct.

The most satisfactory application to the lid in old cases of catarrh is to touch very lightly, and at first very cautiously, the swollen papillæ at the retrotarsal fold with a smooth crayon of sulphate of copper. This is an extremely harsh remedy if applied too freely, and it should not be reapplied under any circumstances until the eye has fully recovered from the first application. As regards internal remedies, I have only to say that the same class is indicated as in the acute form of the disease, and that too brilliant results must not be looked for. We may, however, look for a great deal from

HYGIENIC MEASURES.

In conjunctivitis of all kinds, great attention should be given to hygienic regulations. The sensitive eyes should be protected against bright light during the day or night by plain blue or smoke-colored glasses, which will afford also a measurable protection against wind and dust. The patient should use the eyes with great moderation especially by artificial light, and should particularly avoid all places where the air is necessarily impure, such as crowded rooms like the theatre, lecture-room, ballroom, or rooms where tobacco-smoke prevails. He should be counselled also to avail himself as much as possible of the beneficial influence of a pure out-door air, and should be advised that when necessary to use the eyes in reading, writing, or fine work, preference should be given to the morning hours when the light is constantly growing better.

PURULENT CONJUNCTIVITIS.

Purulent conjunctivitis, which is to be regarded only as a severer and more dangerous form of the catarrhal, is distinguished from the latter by the character and greater abundance of the secretion, the greater swelling of the lids in consequence of the serous infiltration being also sub-conjunctival, the great injection of the sub-conjunctival vessels as well as the increased vascularity of the conjunctiva proper, the chemosis so frequently present, and by the increased size of the mucous papillæ often termed granulations. One of the most practical and certain methods of determining at once whether you have a blenorrhœa or a simple catarrh to deal with, is, by the easy proceeding so long taught in the clinics of Prof. Arlt, of Vienna. The upper lid is to be everted, and if the conjunctiva is sufficiently transparent for us to see the lines of the meibomian glands running towards the edge of the tarsus, we have a catarrh; if the infiltration is so great as to hide these glands, we have no longer a catarrh but either a purulent, a granulated, a diphtheritic, or some graver form of ophthalmia. In purulent conjunctivitis the cornea is much more apt to become involved, and this form is of course more contagious.

THE TREATMENT,

During the inflammatory stage in which there is often considerable fever, must be purely antiphlogistic. Ice-water compresses should be perseveringly used, and these with the perfect quiet of the patient, and the administration of aconite suffice to control measurably the acute symptoms. I have never resorted to the use of leeches, and I have often seen them used in these cases when I thought them unnecessary. If but one eye is attacked, the other should be bandaged as a precautionary measure, and in all cases of purulent ophthalmia the attendants should be warned that the greatest cleanliness and attention to the contagious character of the secretion is necessary for their own safety. After the inflammatory symptoms are subdued, as shown by the diminished swelling of the lids, and the pale red and relaxed condition of the conjunctiva, a cautious use of stimulating collyria is indicated. If the cornea is involved care must be taken that the application does not come in contact with it, by painting it on the everted lids and immediately washing it off as previously directed.

Egyptian, or Military, Ophthalmia is only a variety of purulent conjunctivitis. It was first recognized and named after an unprecedentedly severe epidemic originating in the troops of the English and French armies stationed in Egypt. It spread so fearfully that after the Napoleonic wars England alone had upwards of five thousand blind invalided soldiers to care for. It is doubtful whether this form of the disease is more contagious than any other. Very likely any form of the affection getting a foothold among masses of people crowded together, as in armies, almshouses, and so-called charitable institutions, would spread rapidly. Uncleanliness and bad ventilation are very attractive conditions for this disease. The contagion of a purulent ophthalmia, as is well known, may engender a very light or a very severe form of the affection, — a mere catarrh or a diphtheritis. In the beginning the disease is hardly contagious, but becomes so as it progresses, and the discharge increases in quantity and consistency. The form of the disease produced by contagion seems to depend on local or atmospheric conditions as well as upon the constitution or age of the person infected.

The internal remedies most useful in my practice are zinc, nit. arg., merc., and hepar. The two first in connection with their employment locally, and the two last during the interregnum when stimulating collyria, are temporarily laid aside for the topical use of water or for the remission of all local measures.

CONJUNCTIVITIS IN THE NEW-BORN.

Ophthalmia neonatorum is a purulent conjunctivitis which comes on a day or two after birth. It begins as a very slight discharge, but sometimes increases with great rapidity a few hours later. Its cause is generally to be sought in a gonorrhœal or leucorrhœal discharge of the mother. In mild cases where the discharge is chiefly whitish, not very abundant, and mucous in character, the free use of cold compresses, a careful and frequent removal of the secretion with a soft sponge and tepid water, the administration of aconite and later, puls., merc., or hepar, will suffice to carry the case through to a speedy and successful termination. Such are mild cases. In other instances the affection is severe, and requires prompt and energetic local treatment in order to insure the most favorable results. The responsibility of the physician in a severe case of ophthalmia neonatorum is very great. Intelligent treatment is surprisingly effective, but negligent or unskilful treatment is often deplorable. Our asylums for the blind afford far too many mournful examples of the results of bad treatment in this affection.

TREATMENT OF SEVERE CASES.

If the disease increases in severity in spite of our treatment, we ought never to neglect to determine by fair ocular inspection whether the cornea be intact or not, because upon this circumstance depends the treatment and the nature of our prognosis. It is not a very difficult matter to obtain a view of the cornea even when the lids are very much swollen. The child is to be held by the nurse, its head resting between the knees of the surgeon, and in this position there is generally little difficulty in forcing the lids apart. If the fingers alone are insufficient in consequence of the swollen condition of the conjunctiva, an elevator may be used. It is remarkable how averse many physicians are to this simple procedure, but in no other way can a case be treated so intelligently or conscientiously. It is not at all difficult of accomplishment, and never productive of the slightest injury to the lids. Collyria of alum or sul. of zinc, or injections of these by means of the syringe are often used of the strength of three to five grains of the former or one or two grains of the latter to the ounce of water, but I rarely use them. I prefer a collyrium of nit. of silver, one grain to the ounce of water. It is quite as mild, and I believe vastly more effective. It is particularly indicated when the discharge is copious and wholly purulent. This should be dropped into the eye, after it has been carefully cleansed from the discharge, twice a day. In a few days, if the profuse discharge still continues, and especially if the slightest haze upon the surface of the cornea indicates a complication in this direction, a solution of three to five grains of the nitrate of silver to the ounce, should be painted with a brush upon the everted lids and immediately washed off with tepid water or neutralized by the application of a solution of common salt and water. No evil consequences whatever can result from this proceeding, and not unfrequently the beneficial results of it are seen after a single application. It need not be often repeated. Cold compresses should be employed to lessen the irritation immediately afterwards, and I prefer as internal remedies after aconite in the commencement, mercurius when the discharge is profuse, and the alternation of arsen. with this remedy if the cornea is ulcerated. It is advisable in this as well as all other forms of conjunctivitis, *when there is ulceration of the cornea*, to bandage the eye closely so as to prevent all friction between the lids and the ulcerated corneal surface. I will give the outlines of a case in illustration of this mode of treatment.

Mrs. G., of Boston, brought to me her babe, three weeks old. It had been suffering from purulent conjunctivitis since two or three days from its birth, and, up to the date of her visit, had been steadily growing worse. The physician in attendance had not attempted an examination of the cornea, but had advised her to keep the eyes as free from the discharge as possible, to apply cloths wet in cold water, and had administered small powders internally. The lids were somewhat reddened and swollen in appearance, and considerably puffed up, from the quantity of pus beneath them. After the removal of the accumulated pus, which was accomplished by repeatedly separating the edges of the lids, giving it exit, and wiping it gently away with a soft sponge, wet in tepid water, I was able, without difficulty, by means of an elevator, to open the lids sufficiently to thoroughly determine the condition of the cornea, and make a prognosis as well as diagnosis. The cornea of the right eye was found hazy, and slightly opaque at its upper and inner edge. In the left eye, the corneal opacity was greater; and directly over the pupil was an ulcer, which had already broken through, and occasioned, as I afterwards found, a deposit of matter upon the anterior surface of the capsule of the lens, and a slight adhesion of the free edge of the iris. The mother was informed that the mischief done to the left eye was irreparable; that perfect restoration of sight was impossible; that the disease would probably progress no further, and that vision, to a limited extent, would be preserved to this eye. As to the right eye, there was no question as to its perfect restoration, in every respect. The lids were reversed, and painted with a solution of argen. nit., ten grains to the ounce of water, which was allowed to remain only a second or two, and immediately washed away with tepid water. The nit. argen. was used in an unusually strong solution, because it seemed necessary to check at once, with absolute certainty if possible, further progress of the disease. I have noticed that, when a case is severe, the lids considerably thickened, and the mucous papillæ very much swollen and prominent, it will bear, with good results, and without marked reaction, a much stronger solution of nitrate of silver than it would be prudent or advantageous to apply in a milder case. In this instance, the mother informed me, on her second visit, that the night after the application of the caustic was the best which the child had passed since its birth. There had been no reaction, and consequently no application of cold to the lids had been necessary. Under the circumstances, I concluded to touch the lids a second time with the same solution. This was done on the second day; and again the child had a remarkably comfortable night. On the fifth day, the discharge, which had been very profuse, was considerably lessened in quantity. The mother herself could see a decided improvement, and began to have great confidence in the treatment. I now diluted the solution with an equal part of water, making it five grains to the ounce; and, after a week, it was reduced still more, making it about two grains to the ounce. I had taken the precaution, also, of dropping into the left eye a solution of atropine, two grains to the ounce, in order to draw away the edge of the iris as much as possible from the corneal opening. The application of the solution above described was made but six times, at intervals of forty-eight hours, when the discharge having almost entirely ceased, I gave the mother simply a solution of sul. of zinc, one grain to the ounce of water, to be dropped daily into each eye; and in two weeks from this time the child was well enough to require no further treatment.

Usually it is not necessary nor advisable to use the nitrate of silver nearly as strong as I felt obliged to in this case. I have unbounded faith in the homœopathicity, so to speak, of a solution of nitrate of silver for that diseased state of the conjunctiva in which it secretes *a profuse purulent matter* It should be employed judiciously, and the word judiciously means a great deal in this connection; for probably of all the remedies ever devised for the eyes, this nitrate of silver has, by its injudicious employment during the last twenty-five years, done the greatest injury.

I am very glad to support my views in regard to local treatment of purulent ophthalmias by so good an authority as Dr. Dudgeon, of England. I quote from a case reported in the "British Journal of Homœopathy" for the year 1853, page 361. The case is that of an infant fourteen days old. He says, "It is with great difficulty the lids can be separated so as to obtain a view of the cornea, as the orbicularis muscle everts them and displays a large fleshy mass of inflamed and swollen conjunctiva. The child's general health seems to be unaffected by the disease. I prescribed a collyrium of two grains of nit. of sil. to two oz. of water to be dropped into the eyes twice a day, and for internal use, arg. nit. 6, a dose every six hours." In two weeks the eyes were free from discharge, and perfectly normal in appearance. Dr. Dudgeon then goes on to justify — quoting Hahnemann's authority — the use of local means in the treatment of local diseases generally.

GONORRHŒAL CONJUNCTIVITIS.

Gonorrhœal conjunctivitis, so called, is a variety of this affection associated with a similar discharge from the urethra, through sympathy or extension of the virus over the system, or, as more frequently happens, is caused by direct contact of a urethral discharge with the eye. In the former case, the attack occurs simultaneously in both eyes; in the latter, it commences in one eye first, generally the right, and in its severe form is one of the most rapid and destructive diseases to which the eye is subject. In its mild form the disease resembles a light purulent ophthalmia, and requires similar treatment. In the contagious form, the inflammation is sometimes exceedingly violent. I cannot describe the nature and treatment of this disease better than by giving the main details of a case of a severe type under my care.

CASE OF GONORRHŒAL OPHTHALMIA.

G. L., a young man of seventeen was brought me by his father, Oct. 10, 1868, to be treated for an inflammation of the eyes. The right eye was closed, the upper lid so largely swollen that, at first glance, I thought of abscess. On turning my attention, for a moment, to the other eye the lids of which were but little affected externally, I noticed considerable injection of the vessels of the conjunctiva on either side of the cornea. The affection of the right eye had been noticed first two days previously; but the great swelling had not come on until this morning. The pain was not very severe; the patient, pale and anxious-looking. The lower lid was but slightly distended, and by carefully drawing it downward and away from the upper one which overlapped it, I could see a marked chemosis of the conjunctiva of the globe. There was no doubt about the diagnosis of the case. As the father seemed nervous and apprehensive, however, I concluded to say nothing about its peculiar nature for the moment, telling him simply that the affection was severe, that the left eyelids, on the next day, would probably be very much in the condition presented by those of the right eye to-day; that the boy was not well enough to be out, and that he must be treated in bed. Ice-water compresses to be applied to right eye constantly, and to the left whenever the cold could be borne or felt grateful. Acon. to be taken every hour.

The next morning the external appearance of both eyes was about the same, the upper lids of both being enormously distended. The right was a trifle less sore to the touch, and I was enabled to determine the state of the globe more definitely. The cornea was still intact, but considerably lessened in circumference through the overlapping of the conjunctiva, the chemosis being very great. The conjunctiva bulbi was very red and puffed, looking "like a piece of raw meat." Pulse, one hundred and twenty. Ice-water compresses to be continued night and day. Acon. internally. I now ascertained that the patient had contracted a gonorrhœa three weeks previously. The discharge from the urethra is still rather profuse.

Oct. 12. Externally the swelling of the lids is somewhat lessened, the internal appearance of the eyes the same. The discharge from the eyes is rather thin and flocculent, not such as could be desired. The pain is not severe; pulse about the same; prognosis doubtful. The same treatment to be continued. The sanious discharge to be wiped out from beneath the upper lid with a camel's-hair pencil moistened in warm water, and the edges of the lids to be tenderly cleansed with a soft sponge and tepid water.

Oct. 13. Swelling of the lids much lessened externally. Inflammation is still too acute to admit of caustic application. Appearance of the globe the same, the chemosis being very great. Discharge still watery and slight. Used twice a day a weak solution of carbolic acid in cleansing the inner surface of upper lid. Attendants getting weary and worn in changing the ice-water compresses night and day, I had two little ice-bags constructed and connected by a bridge, like diminutive saddle-bags, to be saddled across the nose, the little bags filled with small bits of ice to rest one over each eye. The upper lid was found still too tender to bear their weight, but a day later they could be borne, and were afterwards used constantly, thereby saving the nurses much labor Acon. merc. internally. The discharge during the next few days became more copious and pus-like, and the external lids became gradually less swollen and red.

Oct. 15. Internal appearance of lids as bad as ever; appearance of conjunctiva bulbi ditto; cornea not fully transparent, that of the right eye quite hazy at its upper third. Raised the upper lids and painted them with nit. arg. five grains to the ounce of water, immediately washing it off with tepid water.

Oct. 16. Treatment continued.

Oct. 17. Considerable pain in the left knee, which I found slightly swollen, and very sensitive to touch. A water compress was applied; pulse, which had fallen to one hundred, now rose again to one hundred and twelve. Acon. and macrot. internally.

Oct. 18. Left knee-joint largely swollen, measuring, with the leg extended, fourteen inches at its largest circumference; sensitive to pressure, and immovable; but less painful than yesterday. Right knee painful, and beginning to swell. Discharge from urethra continues. Eyes much the same in appearance. Cornea of right eye the worse of the two. Prognosis, which had seemed for a few days more favorable, now again doubtful, in consequence of this new inflammation of the knee-joints, which bids fair to reduce the vitality of the patient as it has already his courage, and renders the question as to the power of the cornea to maintain the integrity of its tissues a doubtful one. Upon the solution of this doubt depends the future of the patient. He will be cured in any event, but will his vision be left? I confess that as his knees grew large my hopes grew small. Treatment continued.

Oct. 22. Fever lessened, more appetite, knees less painful, but largely swollen, and the right one immovable. Eyes no better; discharge quite copious. Treatment the same.

Oct. 23. Discovered, this morning, what I had been fearing from the first; viz., ulceration of the cornea. The chemosis having in a measure subsided, the conjunctiva bulbi had receded from the edge of the cornea, which it had previously overlapped, and so uncovered in the right eye a crescent formed ulcer extending nearly around the upper half of its circumference. It was deep, its edges sharp and clean, so that it was necessary to look closely in a favorable light to see its whole extent. An ulcer on the left cornea in nearly the same relative position, not so great in extent, but still ugly and dangerous looking, was discovered also. Both ulcers looked, I thought, as though they were growing larger, therefore without some change in my treatment the right eye would certainly be lost, and perhaps the left one too. I therefore made an immediate change in my treatment. His pulse was one hundred, the tongue was nearly clean, and he had expressed a strong desire for solid food. I determined, if possible, in the present state of his digestive organs, to gratify his wish to the fullest extent. A rare beefsteak was prepared for him at once, and he was to be fed similarly three times a day. Beef-tea was also to be in readiness, so that if he tired of steak it could be substituted for it. He was to have of rare beef at each meal all he desired, with no restrictions whatever. I further substituted for the solution of nitr. argen. which I had been using, one of fifteen grains to the ounce applying it thoroughly to the reflected portion of the upper and lower lids, and immediately washing it away with tepid water. It caused no pain whatever. Merc. and macrot. were given internally.

Oct. 24. Ulcers look no better; knees improving slowly, and can be drawn up or moved slightly without great pain, but are still largely swollen. Patient eats freely of the steak and digests it without trouble; slept better than usual through the night. The discharge from the eyes is rather less: continued treatment; but before the cauterization I dropped a solution of atropine into each eye so as to keep the iris rigid, and as much as possible away from danger in case of rupture of the cornea from the ulceration. After the cauterization the eyes are bandaged sufficiently tightly to prevent movement of the lids. I find the eyes bear this cauterization, repeated every twenty-four hours well, and it has already lessened the discharge.

Oct. 26. Ulceration appears slightly improved, especially in the left eye, where the edges of the ulcer are slightly tinged with yellow, and at the bottom a gelatinous look, as though the reparative process were commencing. Similar indications, but less marked, are also to be seen in the more important ulcer of the right cornea. Patient complains of shortness of breath, which I find is probably occasioned by overtaxing the digestive organs, so I restrict the diet somewhat in quantity, and give nux and bry. for twenty-four hours. Other treatment continued.

Oct. 28. Shortness of breath gone. The eyes are decidedly better. The ulcers are slowly filling up. Discharge from the eyes less. The cauterization now causes quite severe pain, so that ice compresses have to be resorted to afterwards, for a half hour before bandaging. Internally merc. and macrot.

Oct. 30. Eyes improving; knees improving also, but very slowly. The present solution of nit. arg. being now too strong, I reduce it one-half, making about seven and a half grains to the ounce which is borne readily. Discharge from the eyes much less; from the urethra, also, somewhat less. Patient's appetite good, and he is allowed to indulge it in nourishing food, to the fullest extent.

Nov. 6. Improvement in all respects; he manages to walk about the room moderately. Ulcer in the left cornea reduced to a mere trace, that of the right surely but slowly filling up. He can read coarse print.

Nov. 12. Acuteness of vision is nearly perfect, as the opacity left on the cornea from the ulceration, and the reparative process, does not encroach at all on the pupil.

I may mention here that, some three months afterwards, this patient came again under treatment for rheumatic iritis, — a disease of the eye, which often follows gonorrhœal rheumatism. The affection of iris in this instance was only of three weeks' duration.

Merc. internally, and atropine externally, were the remedies used.

Conjunctivitis Diphtheritica is very rarely, perhaps never, seen in this country or in England. It is occasionally epidemic in Berlin. It resembles the preceding in many respects; but is usually more severe and dangerous. The discharge is at first, yellow, thin, and flocculent, the swollen lids rigid from deep-seated fibrinous effusion, the pain and heat very great. In a few days the discharge assumes a purulent character, the lids become less rigid, there may be fibrinous exudation from the conjunctiva, the cornea is very apt to grow hazy and ulceration or sloughing ensues.

The treatment in the beginning should be vigorous. With the greatest care and attention the disease will often terminate unfavorably. Ice and ice-water compresses with aconite until the discharge assumes the character of pus, then the application of a solution of nit. arg. to the lids avoiding contact with the cornea, and the exhibition internally of arg. nit., merc., and arsen. in case of ulceration of the cornea, this, with a generous diet, would be my idea of a treatment which might offer a tolerable chance of saving the eye.

ACUTE CONJUNCTIVITIS GRANULOSA

Is characterized by pain in the eye, photophobia from ciliary irritation, and particularly by the sensation as of a foreign body beneath the lids. If the latter be everted there will be noticed in addition to the swollen papillæ, and intermingled with them, little gray points which are true granulations. After a week or more, the conjunctiva becomes more swollen, the discharge abundant and purulent, and at this stage of the disease it is difficult to distinguish the affection from a conjunctivitis purulentia. This purulent stage continues for some weeks, and may be treated as a conjunctivitis purulentia, exercising great care in regard to the use of irritants. So long as photophobia and lachrymation are marked, no irritating collyria can be used safely. Later, with the exercise of this caution, the affection may be treated like the chronic form mentioned on the next page. *The cause of this affection* is, generally, defective hygienic conditions and contagion. It spreads rapidly, like the military ophthalmia, among masses of people. Either from neglect of all treatment, or from improper or imperfect treatment, or want of persistence on the part of the patient, the disease is very apt to become chronic. The secretion diminishes little by little, the general inflammatory state of the conjunctiva disappears, and the disease concentrates itself beneath the upper lid, and we have a

CHRONIC CONJUNCTIVITIS GRANULOSA,

And generally this is soon supplemented by an affection of the cornea, called pannus.

Pannus is a vascular development in the epithelial layer of the cornea. There is sometimes, but very rarely, an extension of the granulations from the upper lid to the ocular conjunctiva, and thence to the cornea, but generally a pannus is caused by friction and pressure upon the cornea, of the roughened surface of the palpebral conjunctiva, and usually therefore, when we see it, we know, without further examination, that we have a granulation of the lid. These granulations are seated upon the upper lid, mostly upon the reflected portion, and the pannus, of course, is generally found upon the corresponding upper half of the cornea. When later, it has extended downward and encroached somewhat upon the pupil, so that vision is impaired, the patient becomes alarmed, and seeks the advice of the physician. The indication in a case of this kind is invariably to cure the granulated lid. This being accomplished, the pannus disappears of itself.

TREATMENT OF GRANULAR OPHTHALMIA.

The treatment of this class of cases is sometimes difficult and discouraging, owing to frequent relapses; is always prolonged, but, so far as my experience goes, successful. If, as is frequently the case, the patient has suffered for many months or years, has been previously treated unsuccessfully, is gloomy and despondent in anticipation of coming blindness, he should be assured at once that his case is not hopeless; and that, with the proper amount of perseverance on his part, a permanent cure, with a more or less complete restoration of vision, is almost certain. A pannus — something growing gradually over the sight of the eye, and threatening eventually to shut out all vision — is usually a disease of fearful omen to the patient. He comes to the surgeon, also, with great fear and trembling, from the idea that the growth upon the cornea must be cut off. No doubt this view is sometimes imparted by the physician who confounds the growth with that of pterygium. The latter, however is, pathologically, a different formation. The patient then, in the first place, should be rendered as cheerful and hopeful as possible. Hygienic regulations, such as previously mentioned, should be strictly enforced, and above all, the general health, which in these cases is apt to be deficient, must be restored. Without an improved condition of the entire system of the patient through internal medications and the enforcement of salutary rules of living, the most judicious local treatment will be but temporary in its effects. No outline even of internal treatment can be given within the space at my command, as each case must be individualized and treated according to the nature of its deviations from the standard of good health.

As a local means of curing the granulated lid, I employ a smooth crystal of alum, a crystal of sulphate of copper, and occasionally a crayon composed of one part nit. of silver to two parts nit. of potash. Pure nit. of silver in substance I never use, nor do I believe its use ever necessary. I prefer in these old and difficult cases, and use by far the most frequently, a smooth crystal of sulphate of copper. The upper lid being reversed, it is drawn lightly and quickly across that portion of the lid seen to be thickened and granulated, and those portions of the conjunctiva not involved are carefully avoided. Considerable pain will ensue; and, if the patient is very sensitive, it is advisable to apply tepid water or weak salt and water to the conjunctiva the instant after the touch with the caustic. Otherwise, the patient may, after the lapse of a few minutes, if the pain does not cease of itself, bathe the eyes in cold water. Immediately after this application the eye will present a reddened and injected appearance, and should on no account be used until this injection disappears, which will be perhaps in an hour or more. There will also be a feeling of irritation in and about the eye, and until this artificial irritation has fully disappeared, no second application of the crayon should be made. Whether, therefore, the process is to be repeated once in twenty-four, forty-eight, or seventy-two hours, or not oftener than once a week, must depend entirely upon circumstances. Meantime, cold or tepid water may be used freely; simple cerate, if the lids adhere together in the morning, and the administration of constitutional remedies persevered in. In sub-acute cases, where there is considerable secretion, the application of a solution of arg. nit. in water, of the strength of five to ten grains to the ounce, will be useful. It should be painted upon the reversed upper lid, and after fifteen or twenty seconds, neutralized by weak salt and water, from a second brush. Five or ten grains of salt to the ounce is sufficient. After these applications, cold compresses should be freely used until the eye is free from the increased pain.

Pressure is frequently a potent auxiliary in these cases. It can be accomplished by placing a dry compress over the gently closed lids, so arranged that it shall be thickest at the angles, and diminished gradually towards the meridian, in order that the pressure exerted may be as uniform as possible over the granulated surface. An elastic band — flannel makes a good one — is then passed around the head, to hold the compress firmly in its place, and may be drawn as tightly over the eye as can be conveniently borne. This bandage is to be worn night and day, and the compress is to be readjusted upon the eye as often as it becomes in the least displaced.

I will relate a case or two in illustration of the mode of treatment which I find usually so satisfactory.

Miss B., aged twenty-four, visited me first in April, 1865. She complained of irritation and weakness in the left eye, and had recently become much alarmed at the discovery that she could scarcely see to read with it. I found a fully developed pannus extending nearly to the centre of the pupil well supplied with vessels extending downward across the limbus cornea on to its substance. The prognosis, as far as improvement of vision in this eye was concerned, was favorable; *complete* restoration, a sharp, distinct vision like that of the normal eye is very often impossible. The faintest remnant of haziness of the cornea, a cloud upon its polished surface so faint as to be perceptible only by the most favorable lateral illumination will occasion indistinctness sufficient to annoy the patient. When no cloudiness remains, and the cornea regains its perfect transparency, if there is the least irregularity of surface, minute depressions or flattened facets, the rays of light will be abnormally bent in passing through the cornea, and the image upon the retina will be deformed and more or less indistinct. If, therefore, a doubt exists as to a complete restoration of the cornea it is unwise to promise a perfect recovery of vision. The case of this patient was a very old one. In her early youth she remembered an affection of her right eye, and the sight of this eye since, had never been as clear and perfect as that of the left previous to the present attack. On examining the cornea of the right eye by lateral illumination the rays falling obliquely upon the surface, little irregular flattened facets were distinctly seen, which accounted for the lack of sharpness of vision. The lid of the left eye was reversed, and the cause of the growth upon the cornea was found in the granulated state of the conjunctiva. The diseased surface was lightly touched with a crystal of sulphate of copper, very carefully at first, until the eye became somewhat accustomed to the process. Severe pain followed the operation for the first two or three times, but this was effectually controlled by bathing the eye in cold water and immediately going into the open air. This eye had suffered from an acute attack of inflammation as she informed me, more than a year before, but had apparently fully recovered after a few weeks. For a while it continued strong, but gradually grew more and more irritable, until within a few months she had scarcely been able to use it at all without pain. She was under my care nearly five months, and completely recovered. This process of cauterization was repeated on an average about once in three or four days. Mercurius was the remedy principally administered, although she had other remedies for disturbances in her general health during this period. Towards the end of the treatment my attention was called to the benefit of bandaging the eye in similar cases, and she employed this means also with the effect, I think, of hastening the cure. On visiting me nearly two years later, while with the right eye she was unable to read No. 1 type, with the left eye, the one which had been under treatment so long for the pannus, she could read it with ease.

Miss W. came to me first in May, 1867. She also, like the other, was suffering from pannus upon the left eye, and from the same cause. Like the other, also, she had suffered years previously from a probably similar affection in the other eye. The right eye she affirmed had been cured by a doctor in Boston, who had cut the cornea across its upper portion superficially, and had also made longitudinal incisions upon the inner surface of the upper lid. These incisions, she said, were painful, but always afforded her relief, and eventually cured her eye. She wished me to treat her left eye now in a similar manner. I declined her method, and touched the granulated lid lightly with a bit of sul. of copper, but it would not do. After a week I gave up the attempt to touch the granulations at all. The eye was rather the worse for my treatment. The ciliary system of nerves was involved to such a degree that the irritation caused profuse lachrymation and severe and prolonged pain and photophobia. The patient was also of exceedingly delicate and sensitive organization. I therefore gave up temporarily the use of irritants of all kinds. Tepid water was used several times a day, and a compress and bandage, as previously described, was applied, to be worn always at night, and, when convenient, during the day. After two or three weeks there was much less congestion, and the pannus had so far disappeared that the patient could read large print without pain, and with tolerable fluency. I now commenced brushing the granulations beneath the lid with a weak solution of sul. of zinc, which I found could be borne every two or three days. The bandage was continued with great benefit, and during the first part of the treatment, while the eye was irritable, macrotin and spigelia, and later, mercurius were administered internally. After two months' treatment no trace of the pannus was left, and acuteness of vision was the same in each eye.

Aqua chlori is recommended by Graefe for obstinate pannus from granulated lids, and Donders finds two to four parts of olive oil to one of oil of turpentine efficacious. Inoculation of the eye with pus to create an acute purulent inflammation has been more or less successful in desperate cases in clearing up the cornea and restoring vision. *Peritomy*, an operation in which the conjunctiva with its subtissues is excised with forceps and scissors, around the edge of the cornea, I have seen Mr. Bowman, of London, perform with good results. Favorable results, it is said, have also followed the operations of lengthening the palpebral fissure, so as to remove the pressure of the upper lid upon the cornea.

SCROFULOUS CONJUNCTIVITIS OR SCROFULOUS OPHTHALMIA

I place in this chapter, inasmuch as its primary seat is usually the conjunctiva; the cornea, iris, and sclerotica becoming later involved.

DIAGNOSIS.

It is hardly necessary to dwell on the diagnosis. The mere circumstance that ciliary irritation and photophobia so affect the orbicularis that its spasmodic closure nearly renders it impossible to see the eye at all, is of itself an almost unerring indication of the nature of the disease. It is necessary, however, to see the eyeball, in order to determine its precise condition, and form a correct prognosis. A few whiffs of chloroform or ether will sometimes quickly relax the orbicularis; but I prefer a resort to the lid-elevators to be used, as mentioned in Ophthalmia neonatorum. Separating the lids we shall find the palpebral conjunctiva red, swollen, and velvety looking, the ocular conjunctiva injected, the pinkish zone around the periphery of the cornea well marked, the cornea probably dull, opaque, or ulcerated, and the iris perhaps contracted. There is sometimes a good deal of ciliary neuralgia present, and the dread of light may be so intense that the child cannot be induced to turn its face towards the most moderate light even with its eyes tightly closed.

Fortunately the disease is not always of so severe a grade as this, and the photophobia much less severe. In these cases, by means of coaxing, and some little artifice to excite their curiosity, we may, through the exercise of considerable patience, arrive, with most children, at a hasty view of the cornea sufficient for our purpose. Often, the cornea will be found nearly transparent, and the disease confined to the conjunctiva and edges of the lids. Generally, however, even if the cornea appears unaffected, the ocular as well as palpebral conjunctiva is involved, and the inflammation is so deep seated as to reach the vessels beneath the conjunctiva, as shown by the pinkish zone around the edge of the cornea. The irritation of the ciliary plexus of nerves is very great, the eye is exceedingly sensitive to all external influences, there is copious lachrymation and any irritation is followed by most violent reaction. In some chronic cases these symptoms are measurably lessened in severity, but after all a leading characteristic of these cases is the ciliary irritation, and the consequent extreme sensitiveness of the eye. I dwell on this point because of its importance in the treatment.

TREATMENT OF SCROFULOUS OPHTHALMIA.

The treatment of these cases must be almost wholly internal. The disease of the eye is but one of the manifestations of a disorder that pervades the entire system, and topical means can at best be only palliative. Soothing applications, however, like tepid water, milk and water, quite warm fomentations of water, or warm water medicated with belladonna or chamomile or poppy leaves, will frequently quiet a ciliary neuralgia or great restlessness, when internal remedies like bell., cham., coff., or spigel. alone, do not act with sufficient promptness, and should therefore not be overlooked. There are, moreover, some phases of this disease, such for instance as when its chief seat appears to be the edges of the lids, where a mild mercurial ointment, a grain or two of white precipitate, or one grain of red precipitate, to the ounce of lard or cerate, rubbed gently between the cilia, if necessary while the child is asleep, will produce sometimes marvellously favorable results. It should be continued a long time, nevertheless, if we hope for permanent benefit, and merc. should be given internally at the same time. It is customary, I know, at the present time in the "regular" school (so called probably from the regularity with which it changes) to apply an unguent of merc., zinc, lead, or nit. of silver washes to the inner surface of the lids in these cases; but from pretty frequent and continued observation of the treatment in this way in the hospitals of Europe, I am convinced that it seldom does good and very often does harm; and that in homœopathic practice, we may better discard it altogether. An exception to this sweeping condemnation ought perhaps to be made in favor of the mercurial ointment to the inside of the lids, but I do not find its use at all necessary.

This is not the place, nor is it necessary, for me to remark at length on the nature or pathology of what is called scrofula, and its appropriate treatment in general. In the management of these diseases of the eye, hygienic and dietetic regulations are of the first importance. Fresh air, light, warm clothing, and good diet are indispensable always. In regard to light, I do not believe in keeping the patient in a dark room. If there is no ulceration of the cornea, no special attention in a hygienic way need be given in this affection to the patient's dread of light. The celebrated Prof. Beer, who formerly had charge of the department of the general hospital for diseases of the eye during many years in Vienna, used to take children affected with severe photophobia and place them in a position so that the sunlight might fall directly into the eye, and then force the lids apart.

This appears like a very dangerous proceeding, but I have the authority of the grandson of the operator, the present Prof. Ed. von Jäger, to the effect that no injury to the eye or brain was occasioned by the treatment. This kind of procedure, however, is not practised in Vienna at the present time. A rather heroic method, or one which mothers at least would consider so, is practised by Prof. Graefe, in Berlin. When the eyes are much better and yet the photophobia does not yield, he dips the child's head under water, perhaps several times, thoroughly frightening it, and usually with the result of overcoming the spasm of the orbicularis.

When there is an ulcer on the cornea or a vescicle near its edge in the stage of excoriation, the photophobia may arise from the exposure of denuded nerve fibres, and then the progress in reproducing an epithelial covering for the exposed nerves will be very much hastened by bandaging the eye. The bandage will also serve the purpose of preventing friction of the lids in winking, and tend to prevent rupture of the cornea if it happen to be the seat of a deep ulcer. Children also have a disposition to constantly rub their eyes, — a trifling circumstance enough, but one which frequently has seemed to me the chief cause of the continuance of the inflammatory state, — and this the bandage of course completely remedies.

This bandage should be changed several times a day, and the discharge washed from the eye, if discharge be present. Sometimes great pain and restlessness will be promptly relieved by dropping a solution of atropine, one or two grains to the ounce of pure water, into the eye; and its quieting influence seems to expedite the cure. The atropine should never be dissolved in alcohol or alcohol and water, because alcohol applied to the eye is an irritant, and usually contra-indicated in cases where atropine is likely to prove useful as a sedative.

It is almost, or quite, impossible to give even an outline of the treatment that may be required in scrofulous ophthalmia, because, aside from the different tissues of the eye which may be affected, the patient, so far as my experience goes, invariably suffers from general disturbance of the health. A child now under my care, aged eighteen months, has, in addition to the eye trouble, great irritation of brain from the teething process, distension of the abdomen, constipation, loss of appetite, and an appearance of languor. The general status of the child, and especially the constipation, is improving under bry. Possibly opium or collin. might have been as good. With the improved health has come an improvement of the eyes, and yet I cannot say that either of the three remedies mentioned is to be regarded as especially indicated for scrofulous affections of the eyes. The fact is, constitutional symptoms are so generally present, and are so diverse, that almost any remedy of our materia medica may be indicated and prove serviceable to the eyes, through the improvement to the general health, brought about by its administration. It is to be borne in mind that a cure of the eyes is not likely to be permanent unless there is a corresponding benefit to the general health. Hence, local measures need only concern the removal or palliation of the local irritability and pain.

In looking over our homœopathic periodicals, without by any means exhausting them, I find of one hundred and sixteen cases noticed, all of which resulted in satisfactory cures, the following seemed to be the curative agents: merc. in various preparations in thirty-nine cases; sulph. in fifteen cases; calc. in thirteen; bell. in nine; ars. in nine; con. in six; rhus in six; hepar in five; apis in four; silex in two, and a few other remedies in one case each.

Fleischmann, in one hundred and thirty cases treated at his hospital in Vienna, found hepar and sulph. the most serviceable. I doubt the clinical value of general *résumés* like the above, but I presume that there is no doubt that in this affection the remedies above mentioned will be very frequently indicated, and prove very useful. I would add to them spig., and the new American ones, macrot., gelsem., hydras., and baptis. When general symptoms admit, I find myself oftenest giving merc., either vivus or biniodatus, frequently sulph., and when there is corneal ulceration, arsen. Tart. emet. will also prove exceedingly useful in the *photophobia* of scrofulous ophthalmia, and also when herpetic eruptions are present. Dr. Gray reports * some twenty-five cases cured by merc. nit. externally and internally. He uses externally one grain of the merc. to one hundred and fifty drops of water.

PHLYCTENULAR CONJUNCTIVITIS,

Or *herpetic or pustular* conjunctivitis, as it is frequently termed, may be considered as a phase of scrofulous ophthalmia. It occurs usually in children, and mostly in those of a so-called scrofulous diathesis, and very rarely in children otherwise in good health. It is characterized in its simple form by the appearance of a reddened point upon an inflamed base of the conjunctiva, slightly raised, and situated usually either at the limbus of the cornea, or upon the sclerotica, near its junction with the cornea. This red point usually terminates in a vesicle, which, changing into a slight excoriation or ulcer, gradually

* N. A. Journal of Homœop., Feb., 1860.

disappears, and leaves no trace behind. There is generally some irritation of the ciliary nerves, and, as a consequence of this, some photophobia and lachrymation. These symptoms being greatly increased when the vesicle or vesicles happen to come on the cornea or at its limbus. If the vesicles are not developed in too great numbers, and are not too near the cornea, the disease is very slight, and requires very little treatment. I was once consulted, by an adult, in a case of herpetic conjunctiva, whose physician had informed him that he had probably a pterygium growing over the sight of the eye, and it would have to be removed by an operation. He was a sculptor, and I advised him to remain at home for a few days, so as to avoid the dust of his studio, and he was soon cured, without any further treatment whatever. Many cases, however, are much severer than this and not as easily disposed of; and in all the tendency to recur again and again is strongly marked.

TREATMENT

One of the best remedies for this disease is merc. internally, and externally at the same time, powdered calomel. The inspissations of the powder should be made by taking up a minute quantity of the fine powder on a camel's-hair pencil, then holding the pencil vertically before the affected eye, between the forefinger and thumb of the right hand, having exposed the surface of the under lid with the left hand, tap the handle of the brush rather smartly with the ring finger of the right hand, at the same instant tossing the brush slightly towards the lids, and some of the fine dust will be projected directly into the eye. This manœuvre is simple, but it requires a little practice to do it neatly. The calomel should be very fine, but little should be taken up on the brush, and no lumps of it thrown into the eye. Neither should it be blown into the eye through a tube: it is too coarse treatment for a delicate eye, even if well enough for the nose and other parts of the body. The calomel seems to exercise a specific influence in these cases, and cannot be replaced by other powdered substances. For instance, powdered magnesia appears to act simply as an irritant, no curative effect following. I formerly thought the calomel simply an irritant used in this way, but am now convinced to the contrary. It *does* irritate, and should therefore be used cautiously if the eye is very sensitive and dreads the light. For the photophobia, tart. emet. will often be serviceable. Ciliary neuralgia may often be quieted by cham., using at the same time warm fomentations of chamomile water over the closed lids. Generally speaking, the internal remedies will be mostly such as have been mentioned under Scrofulous Conjunctivitis, and directed to the constitutional symptoms so often manifested by an eruption similar to that of the conjunctiva, at the alæ of the nose, angles of the mouth, behind or in the ears, and about other parts of the body.

Sometimes a herpetic point appears in the sub-conjunctival tissue, just at the edge of the cornea. When this is the case, and the sclera or the episcleral tissue is involved, the progress of the disease is tedious in the extreme, and all the more tedious from the circumstance that remedies seem to be of little service. I have had a case of this sort where one vesicle of this kind remained imbedded beneath the conjunctiva for more than three months. It is difficult sometimes in such instances to determine whether such a case should be regarded as a conjunctivitis or an episcleritis. See Phlyctenular Corneitis.

Exanthematous conjunctivitis, occurring during eruptive fevers, does not usually demand special treatment. It is always present to a certain extent in measles, scarlatina, and variola. Any discharge should be removed, and the eyes should be protected against bright light. Bathing in tepid water, or milk and water, is often grateful, and if the edges of the lids adhere, or are tender or excoriated, the application of simple cerate, olive oil, or glycerine will be useful.

Pterygium is a hypertrophied condition of the conjunctiva, usually of a triangular form, the apex towards the cornea, the base at the semilunar fold. The growth is tendinous, and supplied with vessels. If it is not particularly annoying, and does not increase rapidly so as to threaten impairment of vision, by encroaching on the pupillary area, it is better not to disturb it. The operation for its removal is not always permanently successful. A less severe form of the disease consisting merely of a slight hypertrophy of the conjunctiva is readily and successfully removed with the forceps and scissors.

The cause of the disease is usually some injury of the eye or exposure which irritates the conjunctiva, and it sometimes results from a phlyctenular or other ophthalmia. A warm climate predisposes to the affection. For the more pretentious operations for pterygium, I must refer the reader to the larger works on Surgery or Ophthamology.

PINGUECULA.

The little elevation of a yellowish color observed in elderly people at the margin of the cornea, called pinguecula, is not annoying except from its conspicuousness. If desired it may be seized with delicate forceps, and snipped off with the scissors.

Warts of the conjunctiva may be treated in the same way.

Cysts of the conjunctiva are to be treated similarly.

Dermoid tumors, generally seated at the corneal margin, are best dissected out with the knife, care being taken not to go too deeply into the corneal and sclerotic tissues.

CHAPTER VI.

THE CORNEA AND SCLEROTICA.

PHLYCTENULAR CORNEITIS.

THE cornea is frequently the seat of excoriation or ulceration in the herpetic or phlyctenular variety of scrofulous ophthalmia. The objective symptoms are those of herpetic conjunctivitis more strongly marked, with much greater ciliary irritation, congestion, and photophobia. When we meet with a case of scrofulous ophthalmia in which the dread of light is intense, we may be sure that the cornea is implicated. The seat of the vesicle is very apt to be the limbus of the cornea.

TREATMENT.

Arsen. is the most serviceable remedy by far, and comes as near being a specific for this form of corneal ulceration as possible. Tart. emet. frequently acts admirably in the photophobia, and spig. is serviceable for the irritation and redness. Merc., hepar, bell., con., macrot., and gelsem. I also prescribe frequently. To quiet ciliary neuralgia, the instillation of a solution of atropine in water, one grain to the ounce, is very useful, and warm soothing fomentations are also grateful. No irritating applications whatever are to be made to the eye, and a bandage should be applied, for reasons given under the head of Ulceration of the Cornea. After the corneal ulcer or excoriation is healed, and the eye has become less irritable, if the conjunctiva seems to be the primary seat of the affection, as is often the case, powdered calomel, applied as directed under Conjunctivitis Herpetica, will be serviceable, especially in preventing relapses.

ULCERATION OF THE CORNEA.

Corneal ulceration is nearly always an indication of impaired health and weak vitality. There is always more or less congestion of the conjunctiva, and generally pain, lachrymation, and photophobia.

Strumous ulceration, not as the sequence of a vesicle, deeper, and nearer the centre of the cornea, occurs in scrofulous ophthalmia, beginning as an opaque speck. The

Ulceration in ophthalmia neonatorum is similar to this in appearance. A grayish opacity, its centre nearly transparent, the gray then giving place to a tinge of yellow, and this, as resolution sets in, changed again to gray. A blood-vessel or leach of vessels, may often be seen to run from the sclerotic to the ulcer.

Transparent ulcer of the cornea is sometimes observed, in which the vision of the patient, instead of being clouded, suffers only from the irregular refraction of rays of light in passing through the uneven portion of the cornea. All objects appear distorted. The above are generally superficial ulcerations. Among the deep-seated ulcerations, the

Crescentic ulcer of the cornea, as described in the details of the case of gonorrhœal ophthalmia, is one of the more common, while the

Sloughing ulcer, from suppurative corneitis in the weak and ill fed, and the analogous indolent ulcer seen in the aged, frequently complicated by hypopium and suppuration of corneal tissues, are more rarely met in private practice.

THE DANGER

The chief danger of ulceration lies in the tendency to leave a more or less opaque scar or cicatrix in the corneal tissue, and which, if it happen to be situated in or near the centre of the pupillary area, renders vision imperfect. Another danger lies in the direction of a perforation of the cornea, which may occasion a prolapse of the iris, resulting in adhesion between the iris and cornea, displacing the pupil, or distorting it, and perhaps engendering an iritis, or if the perforation happen to be small and central, causing a deposition of matter on the surface of the lens capsule, and forming what is termed a capsular cataract.

TREATMENT OF CORNEAL ULCERATION.

The most potent local agent in promoting a speedy healing of a corneal ulcer is a protective bandage. It is just as essential that the exposed surface of the cornea should be protected from the air, as that any other portion of the body, under similar circumstances, should be covered artificially. The quicker a fresh layer of epithelium is formed to cover the denuded nerve fibres, the sooner will the photophobia vanish. Place a single thickness of fine muslin over the closed eye, then fill the orbit, especially at the inner angle, with fine charpie, so that the band of elastic flannel may press uniformly, but gently, upon the ball of the eye, just sufficiently to prevent winking.

It has been found serviceable sometimes when an ulcer threatens perforation, to anticipate the rupture by puncturing it with a fine needle. The advantage of this is that the opening made is very small and regular, the aqueous humor flows off gently, and the iris falling against the opening, adheres over a very minute surface, and when the aqueous humor once more accumulates, it will be quite likely to be torn away uninjured, and there will remain as a sequence of the disease but a small corneal opacity. Sometimes a perforation has been prevented by a paracentesis of the cornea at its edge, which relieves temporarily the intraocular pressure. In perforation it is of course advisable to prevent the iris being involved, if possible, and to this end the pupil should be kept widely dilated by atropine when the ulcer is situated centrally. If the ulcer is towards the margin of the cornea, it should not be applied; calabar bean may be substituted, in order to contract the pupil as much as possible, and draw its edge away from the seat of the threatened breach.

The diet, in cases of this kind, ought to be as nutritious as the condition of the digestive organs will permit. Fresh meat should be prescribed, and the child should be kept in the open air as much as possible. No darkening of rooms should be permitted; on the contrary the sun should be allowed free access to the nursery, and welcomed as one of the best auxiliaries to the treatment. The dread of light is of course provided for by the bandage, which prevents access of all light, as well as air, wind, dust, smoke, and all deleterious external influences. The heat from the bandage need not be feared; it is beneficial rather than the reverse. In some instances of chronic, indolent ulcerations, heat, either dry or in the form of hot fomentations, is found to hasten a cure admirably. The notion that hot applications soften the corneal tissue, is a fallacy, —there is probably just as much reason for asserting that cold hardens it. The examination of an ulcer on the cornea is much facilitated by *lateral illumination.* This is not feasible when the photophobia is very great, but when it can be resorted to, gives us a correct idea of the depth, extent, and progress of the ulcer. No local applications to the ulcer should be attempted. When the ulceration occurs in the course of a granular or purulent ophthalmia, such applications as are necessary for the cure of the diseased conjunctiva are to be made as previously directed, care being taken that no irritating substance comes in contact with the cornea.

The internal treatment in ulceration of the cornea must be determined to a great extent from the symptoms of the patient apart from those of the eye. I use by far the most frequently arsen., and then merc. and hepar. When photophobia is obstinate or very severe, I frequently alternate with the arsen. either conium, bell., macrot., or tart. emet. The cause of the affection will generally be found in some derangement of the digestive and assimilative functions, and this derangement is the thing, to the removal of which our internal medication must be chiefly directed. I have recently treated in an adult an ulcer of the cornea, following an acute syphilitic affection of the genitals. The cure was speedy and complete under merc. bin. internally, and the use of the bandage and the instillation of atropine, as auxiliaries.

Corneitis frequently occurs in scrofulous ophthalmia, and a similar form of *diffuse corneitis* often complicates a purulent conjunctivitis or a granular state of the lids. It is easily recognized from the hazy, grayish appearance of the corneal surface, and the loss of transparency and polish. Lateral illumination will frequently reveal a minute mottled appearance.

Suppurative corneitis, which is sometimes met with as a result of severe purulent ophthalmia or from chemical or mechanical injury to the eye, or from surgical operations in the corneal tissue, is a much graver form of the disease. It is frequently accompanied by severe ciliary neuralgia. The rose-colored zone around the cornea, contraction of the pupil, and frequently chemosis, are present. We notice a gray opacity, which changes afterwards to yellow as the tissues become broken down, and the end may be a perforation of the anterior chamber. Or there may be extensive corneal abscess, perhaps interstitial infiltration forming onyx. Or a hypopion may result from precipitation of pus to the bottom of the anterior chamber. The matter may reach the anterior chamber from perforation, from extension of the suppurative inflammation to the iris without perforation, or finally from suppuration of the posterior layer of the cornea. Suppurative corneitis is very readily produced by injuries of the cornea in the aged or weak, and is not unfrequently met with as a sequence of typhus, typhoid, cholera, or diabetes.

An indolent or non-inflammatory form of corneitis, where the absence of pain and irritation is a characteristic feature is of still more dangerous nature. The infiltration sometimes extends with great rapidity; and necrosis not only of the whole cornea ensues, but in rare instances the suppuration extends to the entire globe.

TREATMENT OF CORNEITIS.

The treatment of corneitis occurring during the course of the various ophthalmiæ has been sufficiently indicated. In the severe suppurative forms the eye should in the first place be bandaged, and the flannel band should be long enough to pass twice around the head, so that considerable pressure may be exerted on the ball of the eye. Pressure seems to have a controlling influence in limiting the extent of the suppuration, and every hair's-breadth of transparent cornea saved to the patient multiplies infinitely his visual power in the end. If the inflammatory symptoms are so marked as to indicate the cold compress, then the application of the compress bandage may be alternated with the use of cold water. It is hardly worth while to attempt to combine the cold and the compress at the same time. One or the other will be pretty sure to be inefficiently attended to. In the non-inflammatory form of corneitis hot water fomentations of a temperature from ninety to one hundred Fahrenheit are indicated, the object being to create inflammatory reaction. The same treatment for the same object may sometimes be serviceable in the ordinary form of corneitis if the inflammatory appearance is lost and resolution still doubtful. These fomentations are very potent agents for good, or, when indiscreetly used, for evil, and their application should not therefore be intrusted to other than the most trustworthy attendants. When a marked injection of the eye has been induced they should be discontinued, and not again resorted to, unless called for by a recurrence of the former symptoms. It is plain therefore that they should not be used too hot — too long at a time; the cloths should be changed before they become too reduced in temperature, and if too great reaction has been produced it must be neutralized by cold. Paracentesis is sometimes resorted to as a relief from intraocular pressure, to preserve the integrity of the cornea, but very rarely, as of old, for the evacuation of hypopion or interstitial matter.

The instillation of atropine will frequently relieve pain, but if it causes increased irritation, may be replaced by the solution of belladonna, five to ten grains of the extract in pure water.

Aconite, internally, is the remedy to be employed when the reaction is sufficient to warrant the application of cold to the eye, afterwards arsen., for ulceration if it exist, and for the keratitis probably merc. and hepar will be oftenest demanded, although it is quite impossible to forestate what remedies the constitutional symptoms may require. I often recur to cannab., nit. ac., sulph., silex, or in case of ciliary irritation and neuralgia, to macrot., gelsem., spig., con., cactus, nux. vom., and others as intercurrents. Severe pain will usually be relieved if internal remedies fail, by warm medicated fomentations of cham., bell., or opium, administering the remedy also internally at the same time.

STAPHYLOMA ANTERIOR.

Staphyloma of the cornea and iris sometimes occurs as a sequel of perforation or sloughing of the cornea. The iris falls against the opening, lymph is secreted and a cicatricial tissue something of the nature of opaque cornea is formed. Being weak and inelastic under intraocular pressure, it bulges forward, and forms a partial or total staphyloma of the cornea and iris. The disease is to be treated surgically. The intraocular pressure is most certainly relieved by iridectomy beneath that portion of the cornea which still retains transparency, so that the operation may serve at once the double purpose of improving sight and removing pain and disease. This presupposes the staphyloma to be only partial. When it is total the bulging of the eye is so considerable as to present an unsightly appearance; it is irritable, painful, and all sight inevitably lost. All that remains to be done is to remove the staphyloma, not by the old method of excision with the cataract knife and scissors, but after the method of Mr. Chritchett who passes four or five needles armed with fine silk through the base of the growth just behind the line of the contemplated incision, bringing them out at corresponding points opposite; then cutting out an elliptical piece of the cornea within the bounds described by the entrance and exit of the needles, he afterwards draws the needles through and forms a close and even suture. Borelli still more recently practises the removal by strangulation, using two needles which transfix the growth at right angles.

A thread is then passed around the staphyloma behind the pins, and tightly tied, and in three days pins, thread, and protrusion come off together. I have never seen the latter operation performed, but it is said to be particularly successful in partial staphyloma. After the operation an artificial eye may be inserted.

Conical cornea is most readily diagnosed by noting the difference in the size of the image of the window on the two corneæ, or by viewing the eyes in profile. It may also be recognized by the ophthalmoscope. By direct examination we see a central red illuminated space, around this a dark zone, and still outside of this a red ring of light. The dark zone is occasioned by the complete reflection and diffusion of the rays of light at the base of the central cone, where it joins the normal cornea through the periphery of which the outer red ring of light is reflected. One may also get an inverted image of the fundus of the eye, as in myopia, in consequence of the increased refractive power of the centre of the cornea. The bulging is not due to intraocular pressure, for the eyeball is softer rather than harder than in the normal condition. It seems to be due rather to a thinning and weakening of the corneal tissue, the exact nature and cause of which is not well understood. The progress of the disease is generally slow, and this circumstance among others favors the belief that under proper constitutional medication, and favorable hygienic and dietetic influences, the disease might prove curable. I have had no opportunity for lengthened treatment of a case as yet. Ordinarily the treatment is surgical, and by no means entirely successful. The pupil is transformed by the operation of double iridodesis into a narrow slit. This form of pupil neutralizes to a certain extent the astigmatism caused by the unsymmetrical surface of the diseased cornea, by lessening the "circles of diffusion." Some operators, however, prefer a simple enlargement of the pupil by iridectomy towards the peripheral part of the cornea. Graefe sometimes succeeds in flattening the apex of the cornea by producing a minute ulcer upon it, which heals without leaving a permanent opacity. It is a very delicate operation, owing to the extreme thinness of the cornea at this point. Sometimes concave glasses and a stenopaic apparatus with a slit-shaped aperture are useful for the patient in regarding near objects.

Arcus senilis, a line of opacity extending partially or entirely around the periphery of the cornea, caused by fatty degeneration, requires no treatment, as it produces no visual disturbance. It is often hereditary, and sometimes indicates similar disease of other parts of the body.

Opacities of the cornea, resulting from previous disease of its tissue when slight and recent or when dense, the edges not sharply defined, and, in children, usually disappear in course of time without treatment.* Appropriate medical and hygienic treatment will, however, hasten this result. Internally, calc., cann., hepar, merc., sulph., silex., puls. nutt., and other remedies are accredited, and probably justly, with having removed such opacities. The remedy must be selected often according to other irregularities apart from those of the eye. When there are no irregularities in the general condition of the patient's health to guide us, and the eye is not abnormally sensitive, we may try the cautious use of irritating collyria. One or two grains of sul. of zinc or sul. of copper, ten or twenty grains of borax, three to five grains of iod. of pot. each to an ounce of water are sometimes useful. In these cases atropine should be occasionally used to diminish intraocular pressure, and promote absorption. I have used powdered calomel daily with satisfactory effect, as directed in phlyctenular conjunctivitis, and sul. of soda is recently recommended, to be brushed with a camel's-hair pencil over the conjunctiva of the reversed upper lid. Whatever agent we may use to promote local reaction

* Fresh opacities of the cornea are a much greater disturbance to vision than old ones of the same size and apparent density.

it should be changed often, as the eye soon becomes accustomed to the same irritant, and is no longer favorably affected by it. It is hardly necessary to remark that none of those local irritants are admissible until after all inflammation of the cornea has disappeared.

When an opacity is old, and has assumed a white, pearly, glistening appearance, its margin well defined, and especially if in an adult, we shall fail in any attempt to remove it either by internal or external means. We have then the resource of an artificial pupil, to be made exactly behind such part of the cornea as retains most of its normal transparency.

Nussbaum, of Munich, some years since, tried the plan of removing the central portion of an opaque cornea, and inserting a circular window of glass. It was not successful; suppuration and expulsion of the glass followed. The operation of transplantation of cornea has also failed. It is always melancholy to see, and saddening to be obliged to tell, a patient the interior of whose eyes is perfect and who could see, if only the foggy cornea could be replaced by some transparent medium, that there is no hope left for him. It is not unreasonable to believe, I think, that the future of surgery will provide some remedy more or less complete for these unfortunates.

EPISCLERITIS.

Episcleritis commences in the form of a dusky-red circumscribed spot, beneath the conjunctiva in the episcleral tissue or superficial tissue of the sclerotic, generally near the edge of the cornea. As it progresses the color usually changes to a purplish hue. It causes a good deal of ciliary irritation and neuralgia if it involves the edge of the cornea. Otherwise there is little or no pain and little injection of the conjunctiva. It is of not unfrequent occurrence in the course of a scrofulous ophthalmia, and is then accompanied by a conjunctivitis and perhaps some mucous discharge. It must not in these cases be confounded with a pustular or phlyctenular ophthalmia. No ulceration or excoriation ensues, but the spot or nodule gradually pales away.

The cause of the affection when idiopathic is generally debility from overwork, or some depressing influence. It is not difficult to relieve or cure when the patient can be thoroughly under control. Warm fomentations are always soothing, and atropine when necessary will quiet the ciliary neuralgia which is apt to come on at night. All use of the eyes is to be prohibited, and a shade worn when in the open air. Constitutional disturbances will frequently indicate the choice of internal remedies, otherwise I rely almost wholly upon the protiodide of mercury, which in my hands has seemed to be very serviceable. Next to this remedy bry. especially in sudden redness and irritation in the course of the disease, brought on by overuse of the eye.

An unnatural bulging of the sclerotic often occurs as the result of old choroiditis or irido-choroiditis. It is not unusual in cases of glaucoma. It is situated commonly at the anterior part of the sclerotic behind the ciliary region, and is called frequently *anterior staphyloma* in distinction to a posterior staphyloma of the sclerotic seen in progressive myopia. The disease is not idiopathic, but supervenes upon inflammation of some portions of the uveal tract, and presents no characteristic features except in the bulged and bluish appearance of the thinned sclerotic. The treatment will be directed to the iris, choroid, or ciliary body. Sclerotico-choroiditis posterior is noticed under Myopia.

CHAPTER VII.

THE IRIS.

HYPERÆMIA OF THE IRIS

PRESENTS symptoms similar to those of simple iritis, except that they are less marked and the exudation is absent. It may be caused by over-exertion of the eyes for near objects, and often indicates a congestion of the deeper seated structures of the eye. It is frequently noticed in scrofulous ophthalmia, and is not unfrequently one of the results of an injudicious use of caustics. The treatment will depend upon its course, and the nature of the associated affection. Generally it will require a treatment similar to that for iritis.

SIMPLE IRITIS, OR RHEUMATIC IRITIS.

The objective symptoms are injection of conjunctiva, also subconjunctival injection, the rose-colored zone around the cornea being well marked; generally there is contraction of the pupil and always sluggishness in dilation and contraction, discoloration, a blue iris becoming greenish, and a brown iris reddish-brown, and there may be observed frequently a plastic exudation at the pupillary edge or on the surface of the iris. In severe cases there is sometimes swelling of the lids, injection of the conjunctiva, chemosis and the posterior surface of the cornea may be mottled by minute depositions of lymph. The subjective symptoms are sometimes merely dimness of vision and slight dread of light. At other times we find them very severe; there is great pain in the eyeball, around the orbit, and in the temple, generally worse at night, severe photophobia and lachrymation.

SUPPURATIVE IRITIS,

The symptoms of which correspond generally to those above given, is a deeper seated form of inflammation, the tissues of the iris being attacked and becoming swollen and thickened. This is the form which a syphilitic iritis usually takes, while the rheumatic form, so called, when it occurs in rheumatic subjects, is a simple iritis. In suppurative iritis the exudation is copious, the swollen tissues of the iris impede circulation, the vessels become congested, and soon large tortuous veins appear on the face of the iris. Observation by lateral illumination will be of great help in noting the structural changes which occur. Little yellowish nodules may be seen about the edge of the pupil, the mischievous purpose of which seems to be to stick the edge of the pupil firmly to the capsule of the lens. The aqueous humor becomes increased in bulk, and turbid from the admixture of pus and lymph thrown out by the iris. The latter is sometimes completely covered by a thin veil of exudation so as to be quite indistinct, and the exudation may be so extensive as to settle to the bottom of the anterior chamber, forming a hypopium. In syphilitic iritis there are also frequently the tuberculous nodules on certain portions of the iris, reddish-yellow in color, and which attain often to considerable size, and may even project so far into the chamber as to touch the posterior surface of the cornea. I never saw these condylomatous nodes in a non-syphilitic case; such instances have, however, been observed; but, generally speaking, these nodes determine the nature of the case at once.

A SEROUS IRITIS

Is observed generally in children with the peculiar notching of the incisors which indicates hereditary syphilis. There is increased secretion of the aqueous humor which is turbid, and deposits small specks of lymph upon the posterior surface of the cornea; hence the affection has been called *keratitis punctata*. It is frequently associated with choroiditis, and the prognosis is not as favorable as in most other forms of iritis.

THE CAUSE OF IRITIS

Is frequently the exposure to changes of temperature, cold rain, wind, and like influences. The same causes which tend to develop a rheumatic attack, often occasion this, and it is then as well as at other times often called rheumatism of the eye or rheumatic ophthalmia. The pain in this form often extends over the whole of one side of the head and face, and the patient is apt to suffer from relapses. It is frequently of traumatic origin, and frequently of syphilitic. Most cases of idiopathic iritis in children are probably of syphilitic origin. A chronic iritis, though not very often seen apart from a choroiditis, may supervene upon an acute attack. The prognosis of iritis when seen in the beginning, before extensive adhesions between the iris and capsule of the lens have formed, is very favorable. Adhesions almost preclude the possibility of a permanent cure, unless they can be overcome. The edge of the pupil once firmly glued to the capsule, the iris is for ever being irritated by the efforts of the pupil at dilation and contraction, and this irritation constantly tends to produce a sub-acute attack of iritis, and may finally lead to irido-choroiditis and loss of sight.

THE TREATMENT.

The treatment should in the first place look to the prevention of these adhesions by the enlargement of the pupil to the full extent by atropine. For this purpose it should be used of the strength of four grains to the ounce, and be dropped into the eye at intervals of five minutes three or four times, morning, noon, and night. Less frequent use than this will sometimes keep the iris dilated to its maximum, but not always. In mild cases a drop or two once a day will often suffice. Another benefit of the use of atropine is, that it gives the inflamed muscular tissue of the iris perfect rest through the complete paralyzation of the constrictor pupillæ. Otherwise, the iris is in constant motion attempting to regulate the size of the pupil according to the nature of the light. An inflamed muscle in any other part of the body we should hardly attempt to cure, unless we could first be certain of the condition of rest being fulfilled. Another advantage of the atropine also is, that the intraocular pressure being lessened by its use, as shown by diminished tension (hardness) of the eyeball, interior circulation is relieved and the congestion of the iris and ciliary body is lessened.

Sometimes recent adhesions have been broken up quickly by the alternate use of a solution of atropine and calabar bean, thus producing extreme alternate dilation and contraction of the pupil.

For internal medication I rely chiefly on acon., bell., merc., and bry. Acon. at the commencement, particularly when the pupil is much contracted, with bell. in alternation, or bry., if in a rheumatic subject. Severe pain in the eye and about it is often relieved by warm fomentations medicated or unmedicated, and the administration of spig., cham., macrot., gelsem., or other remedies, according to special indications. Merc. will often be serviceable for pain, especially when aggravated at night. I have recently been treating a case of iritis, following an attack of rheumatism with bry. and merc. in alternation. Atropine twice a day served to keep the pupil sufficiently enlarged and to quiet the neuralgia. A case of syphilitic iritis, showing the characteristic nodules on the iris, very severe, with great exudation, great tension of the ball, and severe ciliary neuralgia, so that I thought strongly of a paracentesis corneæ to relieve the two last symptoms, recovered perfectly, leaving no adhesions, under atropine, warm fomentations and the internal use of acon., merc., and later, when I found a tendency to complication of the choroid, kali hydriod. It is much safer in treating iritis, even if not very severe, to confine the patient to the house, and to the bed, if the attack be important. The darkened room will not be so necessary if atropine be used, still in all cases it will be more agreeable to the patient to have the bright yellow light moderated to a certain extent. When necessary for the patient to go out, he should wear a blue or green shade. In chronic iritis, when adhesions are left and irritation of the iris is kept up by them, a strong solution of atropine being of no avail in breaking them up, the operation of Corelysis may be indicated. After ascertaining the exact position of the posterior synechiæ by lateral illumination, a small incision is made through the cornea with a needle, and a blunt hook, called, from its form, a spatula hook, is introduced, and the adherent iris separated from the lens. The great danger in this procedure, as indeed in all operations on the iris, lies in the difficulty of avoiding the rupture or incision of the capsule of the lens.

A chronic iritis, or *irido-choroiditis* may, sometimes be mistaken, at first, for a glaucoma; the diagnosis is readily corrected in such an event by testing the extent of the field of vision. If glaucoma is present we shall generally find it limited. *Choroido-iritis* is an affection primarily of the choroid, the iris being involved secondarily. The prognosis in the latter is more unfavorable; for while in the former an obscurity of vision may be due to a deposition of matter or pigment upon the capsule of the lens, in the latter it is due to changes in the deeper structures of the eye. The medical and hygienic treatment of these cases will be that of iritis and choroiditis.

PROLAPSUS OF THE IRIS

Frequently occurs from perforation of the cornea from ulceration or otherwise. If slight, we may succeed in replacing it with a delicate probe, or by enlarging the pupil with atropine, it may be pulled away from the gap. In any event the eye should be covered by a firm compress bandage, to prevent increase of the protrusion. If the prolapse is rather large and bulged outward from the aqueous humor it should be pricked with a needle, causing it to shrink and dwindle away gradually. It may sometimes be necessary, after pricking it, to prevent its refilling, to cut it off with scissors close to the cornea. It should never be touched, according to the custom of many surgeons, with caustic, as it causes great iritation, and may set up an iritis, and because under any circumstances it is quite an unnecessary risk to run.

CYCLITIS.

Cyclitis, or irido-cyclitis may arise from a severe form of iritis in which there is an irrepressible tendency to cell proliferation, so that the disease soon reaches the ciliary bodies, or from injury of the eye. The inflammation in the ciliary body, when not idiopathic, corresponds in character to the nature of the iritis from which it originates. It is recognized by the tenderness of the eyeball to touch in the ciliary region, and it is generally the occasion of a good deal of ciliary neuralgia. Its treatment in the main is that given for iritis. It may arise also from the extension forward of a choroiditis, and would then require the treatment principally of a choroiditis. It is always a serious complication, and our prognosis should be guarded. It is noticed further under Sympathetic Ophthalmia.

ARTIFICIAL PUPIL.

The formation of an artificial pupil is indicated when the natural one has become closed by disease, and also, when the pupil being normal or otherwise, the cornea has become opaque to a certain extent, but has still a transparent portion left. Behind this transparent bit of cornea exactly, the new pupil must be made. Or, if the cornea be transparent over considerable of its surface, we enlarge or extend the natural pupil in a direction which will render it most serviceable to the patient. Other things being equal, the extension of a pupil downward and inward is best for vision.

The operation usually is that of iridectomy, the same, with an important exception, that of the location of the incision, as the iridectomy made for the relief of glaucoma, or intraocular pressure. A small incision is made into the cornea near the point beneath which we desire the new pupil. This incision is made generally with a keratome — a lance-shaped knife. If a gush of aqueous humor has not already prolapsed the iris we enter the anterior chamber with a pair of delicate forceps, and grasping a portion of the iris near the incision, draw it through the wound and snip it off with a pair of curved scissors.

A narrower and sometimes better pupil, optically considered, is sometimes formed by the operation of iridodesis. The incision is made at the edge of the cornea with a broad needle. The chamber is entered with a blunt hook, and the iris caught between its pupillary and ciliary edge, and drawn through the wound, around which has previously been placed a fine loop of silk. The portion of iris drawn out is ligatured with the silk, and in the course of a few days sloughs off. A double iridodesis is frequently performed in opposite directions which gives a narrow slit for a pupil like that of a cat. This is the operation usually done for conical cornea. When the anterior chamber is very narrow, the slender cataract knife of Graefe may be used instead of the lance-shaped keratome, in order to avoid the risk of wounding the capsule of the lens. The opening is made along the rim of the anterior chamber, as in the flap operation for cataract, only shorter.

Iridodialysis is not so formidable an operation as its name would indicate. It is simply entering the anterior chamber with a hook or forceps, and tearing away a part of the iris from its ciliary attachment. This forms a pupil, which answers when only a narrow line of the cornea at its periphery is transparent.

Artificial pupil by incision simply, with a broad needle, may be performed for a pupil entirely closed, when there is no lens, as after cataract operation. After the puncture, the fibres of the iris, if it is tolerably healthy, will retract sufficiently to form a pupil; if not, a bit of the cut edge of the iris may be drawn out at the small aperture in the cornea and excised with the scissors. A much more difficult operation, that of excising a triangular piece of iris with delicate scissors is sometimes resorted to under similar circumstances.

AFTER-TREATMENT IN THESE OPERATIONS

May be very simple. A bit of linen is laid over the closed lids, the orbit filled out with a little charpie, and a light bandage applied, and for forty-eight hours aconite may be administered hourly when the patient is awake. It is rarely necessary to resort to the cold compress.

MYDRIASIS

Is the name given to a state of the pupil when abnormal dilatation and more or less immobility are present. It is a well known symptom, when binocular, of grave diseases of the brain. It is generally however of much less serious import, and may follow a rheumatic attack from exposure to cold or wet. It follows upon partial or complete paralysis of the third nerve, and is often of syphilitic origin. A very common extra-ocular cause, according to my experience, is irritation of the sympathetic, from disorder of the digestive organs, spinal irritation, or, in children, helminthiasis. Monocular, as well as binocular, it is often owing to deep-seated diseases of the eye, which, by diminishing the sensitiveness of the retina, impair the reflex action upon the ciliary nerves which control the pupil. It frequently follows injury of the eye. I have lately had under my care a man who, while cutting wood, was struck not very forcibly on the ball of the right eye by a splinter. No wound or discoloration occurred, but the pupil immediately enlarged, and has, up to the present time, some two months, not regained its former contraction. Occasionally I have had a case of monocular dilatation of the pupil from over-exertion of the eye.

This is to be explained probably by the fact that the eyes differed slightly in refractive power, and the affected eye did most of the work. The affection occasionally follows injury of the sphincter of the pupil from pressure of the lens in extraction. A constant subjective symptom is the impairment of vision for near objects.

I cannot define any particular plan of treatment. It must vary constantly according to the nature of the exciting cause. The affection is often a concomitant of paralysis or disease of other parts of the eye, and the treatment, is spoken of elsewhere. Calabar bean applied to the eye is generally of temporary benefit in restoring the size of the pupil, and improving the vision for near objects: the same remedy is reported occasionally to have been of permanent benefit also.

MYOSIS,

The opposite of the above condition, an abnormal contraction of the pupil, is sometimes seen in iritis, and frequently in disease or injury of the upper part of the spinal cord. It has also been observed in hyperæthesia of the retina and in persons who work at small objects, like watch-makers. Idiopathic myosis is extremely rare.

Congenital anomalies of the iris occasionally observed are *iriderемia*, absence of the iris, *coloboma*, or cleft iris, *corectopia*, an eccentric position of the pupil, and *polycoria*, more than one pupil.

ACTION OF ATROPINE AND CALABAR BEAN.

Atropine, to be used in the form of a solution of sulphate of atropine, which is exceedingly soluble in water, acts on the iris principally by paralyzing the circular fibres, but also by contracting the radiating fibres. The iris is extremely susceptible to its influence, a solution in water of $\frac{1}{10,000}$ enlarging the pupil, which it reaches by absorption through the cornea, with great certainty, in the course of an hour or two. The disadvantage of a weak solution lies in its feebleness in overcoming any adhesions between the iris and capsule of the lens, and also in its uncertainty of effect when the iris is diseased. For the enlargement of the pupil when the iris is healthy, a weak solution, such as a grain to ten or twelve ounces, is preferable, from the fact that its effect passes off in the course of a day or two. A solution of a grain or two to the ounce of water, is often desirable on account of the promptness of its action, a half hour only being required for its full effect. A solution of four grains to the ounce will act still more promptly, and will be certain also to completely paralyze the accommodation when this is desirable; the effect of such a solution will not pass wholly off for eight or ten days. A solution two or three times this strength may be used in attempting to break up old adhesions between the iris and lens capsule. Very strong solutions, thirty to fifty grains, are not to be commended, lest cerebral symptoms supervene. A long continued use of atropine renders the eye intolerant of it, and in very rare instances it proves too great an irritant to be used at all.

CALABAR BEAN.

The calabar bean (*Physostigmatis Faba*) appears to exercise on the eye an effect exactly antagonistic to that of atropine. It contracts the pupil, rendering the eye temporarily myopic. Its effects are more rapid and less permanent than those of atropine, and as with the latter, are more rapid and permanent, the stronger the solution made use of. The usual strength is that of about four grains to the ounce of water. It will neutralize the action of atropine to a certain extent, restoring the pupil to its natural size, but the effect is evanescent, passing off in a few hours, when the pupil again enlarges, the atropine resuming its control.

Iridodonesis, tremulousness of the iris, is a certain indication that the iris has lost the support of the lens, as after extraction, in dislocation of the lens, or as in hydrophthalmia, when the anterior chamber becomes enlarged.

Cysts of the iris, may be excised together with that portion of the iris to which they are attached, by the operation of iridectomy.

CHAPTER VIII.

THE CHOROID AND VITREOUS.

HYPERÆMIA OF THE CHOROID

Is undoubtedly of frequent occurrence, but is very difficult to diagnose with the ophthalmoscope as the vessels of the choroid are, except in very light-complexioned persons, almost completely hidden by the pigment layer. Nor unless the iris and ciliary bodies are also congested does it seem possible to diagnose it without the ophthalmoscope. When its existence is determined, and it may always be suspected in hyperæmia of the retina, if venous or passive in character, ham., externally and internally, should be used. See Treatment of Hyperæmia of the Retina and of the Conjunctiva.

CHOROIDITIS SIMPLEX, OR DISSEMINATED CHOROIDITIS,

Can hardly be diagnosed with certainty without the aid of the ophthalmoscope, as the otherwise noticeable symptoms are common to other affections. There is usually some dilatation and sluggishness of the pupil, some failure of sight, irregular obscuration of the field of vision, so that perhaps but parts of objects are seen at once, and usually little or no pain. Sometimes the external appearance of the eye is quite normal. The

Ophthalmoscopic signs are general cloudiness of the choroid or vitreous, but oftener we see small yellow-white patches of lymph, first at the periphery, afterwards about the macula lutea and optic disc, and later, if atrophy of the choroid occurs, the white sclerotic will be seen shining through in spots. White patches with a pale-red zone around them indicate a syphilitic origin of the disease. Still later, we may find consecutive atrophy of the retina and optic nerve. We know that the exudation at first is in the choroid from the observation that the retinal vessels are distinctly seen over these patches, and are not interrupted in their course or obstructed, and from the fact that the retina retains its normal transparency.

The prognosis must of course be guarded owing to the tendency to complication and atrophy of the retina and optic nerve. Sometimes, however, the exudations are absorbed, leaving but faint traces of their existence behind, and sight is quite restored.

THE TREATMENT

Must be governed to a great extent by the state of our patient's health otherwise, and the cause of the disease. This is frequently syphilis. Generally it will be found that the liver, digestive organs, or the uterus, are disordered. All these circumstances will influence our treatment. At all events, the patient should abstain from the use of the eyes in reading or sewing, and guard them against bright light out of doors by wearing blue glasses. I have more faith in the administration of merc. than in that of any other one remedy, for this disease, and for affections of the choroid generally. No doubt ars., iod., sulph., kali hydriod, or bell., cactus, con., nux., spig., and many other of our remedies, may prove useful in choroiditis. My experience has not enabled me to fix upon definite and reliable indications for the selection of one of these drugs in preference to another, as far as eye-symptoms are concerned. I would give the first group in connection with mercury; the second, occasionally with the first, in irritability, congestion to the choroid and retina, and in photophobia.

In old cases of irido-choroiditis the operation of iridectomy will frequently be indicated for the purpose of breaking the adhesions between the lens capsule and iris, as well as for the purpose perhaps of laying a pupil before a transparent portion of the capsule. The operation is, under these circumstances, beset with difficulties from the narrowness of the anterior chamber and the degenerated rotten condition of the iris. If the lens is wounded in the attempt, it must be extracted. In these cases some operative interference is necessary, as no medicines can be of avail so long as the irritation is kept up by the adhesions. These adhesions may generally be detected at once by the use of atropine; unless the entire pupillary margin is adherent, the enlarged pupil will be irregular in form.

SUPPURATIVE CHOROIDITIS,

Called also *panophthalmitis*, or *ophthalmitis*, is a very grave disease and its course often very rapid. The eyelids are usually red, swollen, and œdematous, the chemosis very great, so that the eye appears swollen. The iris is bulged forward and discolored, the eyeball sensitive to touch, the tension increased, and we notice, if the pupil is sufficiently clear, a yellow reflex from behind the lens, due to a purulent infiltration of the vitreous. Sometimes the pain in the eye and the region about is of the most intense nature, at other times less severe. Sight is, of course, rapidly and greatly impaired, and frequently all sensation of light disappears.

The causes are suppurative inflammation of the iris and cornea in bad subjects, typhus, typhoid, pyæmia, injuries of eye, surgical operations, or sympathetic ophthalmia.

THE TREATMENT OF OPHTHALMITIS

In the commencement should consist of ice-water compresses and the internal use of acon. It may be necessary afterwards if hot fomentations and the administration of the indicated remedies do not relieve the severe pain, to resort to the subcutaneous injection of morphia in the temple, or what is perhaps still more efficacious generally, the paracentesis of the cornea. If the febrile symptoms will permit, the patient should be allowed a most nourishing diet, and perhaps a tolerably free use of stimulants. It is of course often impossible to save the sight of the eye, and indeed frequently any part of the eyeball, in these cases, but unfortunately it has not been considered safe always to remove the eye in panophthalmitis lest the suppurative process extend to the brain. When the disease is foreseen and before the suppuration has become general, enucleation of the ball is probably the best course to pursue. Recently the operation has been frequently performed during the suppurative stage, and no harm to the brain has ensued. Perhaps no danger is to be apprehended unless the brain be previously affected.

Tubercles of the choroid have been detected by the ophthalmoscope. They are seen as small circular rose-colored or gray-white spots mostly in the neighborhood of the optic disc. The disease coexists with acute miliary tuberculosis. The vision is generally normal. Tumors, ossifications, carcinoma, and sarcoma are met with in the choroid occasionally, but they are comparatively rare.

HYALITIS,

Or inflammation of the vitreous humor, though usually an accompaniment of disease of other structures of the eyeball, may nevertheless occur idiopathically. In simple hyalitis we notice with the ophthalmoscope that the whole vitreous is clouded so that the details of the fundus are indistinct, while floating about in it are discovered delicate shreds of various size and shape. Generally with this form of hyalitis there coexists a retinitis, choroiditis, or cyclitis.

A suppurative hyalitis supervenes upon suppurative iritis or irido-choroiditis, and occurs after cataract operations and injuries of the eye, and is sometimes but the beginning of an ophthalmitis which destroys the entire globe. The treatment of hyalitis must have reference to the primary seat of the disease, which is in the choroid or retina. I have never met with it in its idiopathic form.

Opacities of the vitreous are frequently due to remains of effusions of blood or lymph, degenerated fatty or pigmented cells, membranous débris of various form and size. These opacities may be seen with the ophthalmoscope in the upright image best. Let the patient turn his eye in different directions in quick succession and the opacities will be noticed moving slowly about across the pupillary field. Such opacities must not be confounded with the phenomenon called *muscæ volitantes,* usually a physiological condition.

Muscæ volitantes are either transparent or opaque, and are best seen by looking towards a white surface. They are probably caused in most cases by overuse of the eyes, and consist of the débris of cells, shreds of tissue or fibre floating about in the vitreous, and slowly changing their position with every movement of the eye. They appear transparent and bead-like, or in other cases shred-like or as dark queer shaped bodies. Rest of the eyes should be enjoined, the general health attended to, and, if very troublesome, blue glasses may be worn which will render them less apparent.

Hemorrhage of blood into the vitreous is not very uncommon, either from disease of the coats of the vessels, or as a result of a traumatic injury to the choroid. It is sometimes distinguishable by a red reflex, with the ophthalmoscope; at other times the fundus is completely darkened, and cannot be lighted up.

THE TREATMENT OF OPACITIES OF THE VITREOUS

Must be directed to the removal of the cause, which will generally be found to be an irido-choroiditis, or choroido-iritis, or some affection of the deeper structures of the fundus. I see no reason why ham. should not prove an excellent remedy in diseases of the choroid affecting the venous coats particularly, and to this might be added arn., phosph., arsen., caust., sulph., and other of our remedies. Occasionally fixed opacities of the vitreous have been torn through with a fine needle, and the visual powers of the patient improved by the operation.

Synchysis is the name for a fluid condition of the vitreous, in which its gelatinous consistency is lost. It is difficult to diagnose with certainty in all cases. The free movement of opacities presupposes it, and when vitreous is lost from a wound or during an operation for cataract, we know that its loss is made good by a fluid or serous substance. *Sparkling synchysis* expresses a state of fluid vitreous holding crystals of cholesterine, which present a very striking and characteristic appearance under the ophthalmoscope. Their origin or mode of production is undetermined.

CYSTICERCI IN THE EYE.

Graefe has had, in eighty thousand patients, eighty cases of cysticerci in the vitreous or retina:

three cases in which it was in the anterior chamber; beneath the conjunctiva, five; and in the lens and orbit, one each. The result, when the cysticercus is deep seated, is the loss of the eye from inflammation, and degeneration of the choroid and vitreous. Von Graefe has occasionally succeeded in saving the eye through the extraction of the parasite, but the operation is very difficult when the animal is seated behind the lens. The original seat of the cysticercus is usually beneath the retina, where it may be seen with the ophthalmoscope as a grayish-blue vesicle, and from whence it emerges later into the vitreous.

CHAPTER IX.

GLAUCOMA.

THIS is one of the most dangerous of all the diseases to which the eye is subject, and, without timely surgical interference, generally terminates in blindness, and, later, in complete degeneration of all the tissues of the eye. It is not a new disease, but up to the time of the invention of the ophthalmoscope it was not much understood. No remedies, surgical or other, having proved of much avail, it was quite natural that an almost uniformly fatal disease, of which very little in regard to its nature was known, should receive less attention than others better understood, and which permitted of satisfactory alleviation or cure. In 1854, Ed. von Jaeger, soon followed by Von Graefe, gave accurate descriptions of the morbid changes in the fundus occurring in the course of the affection, which drew attention to the disease, the interest in which was widely and quickly spread over Europe when Von Graefe, in 1856, discovered a successful surgical remedy for it in the operation of iridectomy. Perhaps the most convenient and practical way in considering the disease is, to divide it into three forms, — the acute, sub-acute, and chronic.

THE PREMONITORY SYMPTOMS

Of acute glaucoma are usually, first in order, an increased tension (hardness) of the eyeball. This is to be determined by touch, as previously described. The subjective symptom of fulness and swelling, so often felt in conjunctivitis, iritis, or scleritis, is not to be mistaken for increased tension of the ball which indicates the approach of an acute attack of glaucoma. With this tension come its first legitimate fruits, periodic dimness of vision, such as one may produce by pressure of the finger upon the normal eye, lasting for a few moments or hours, and a rapid development of any previously existing presbyopia. The pupil is somewhat, but not greatly, dilated; and as a sequel of this there is constantly noticed by the patient a halo or rainbow around a candle. The ring around the light is at its outer side red; its inner, bluish-green. There may be more or less ciliary neuralgia over the eye, in the forehead, temple, and face; but in my experience this symptom at this time is very apt to be absent. The above premonitory symptoms are all observable without the use of the ophthalmoscope, and may occur merely at intervals of months; but gradually the intervals shorten, and only weeks or days intervene between the recurrence of the symptoms, and the next stage of the disease, *confirmed glaucoma*, may be looked for.

Hereafter, though there are to be perhaps periodic exacerbations, there are not to be, as in the premonitory stage, any *perfect intermissions.* The patient may be suddenly seized with a terrible neuralgia over the eye, in the forehead, temple, face, down the side of the nose, with severe constitutional symptoms, high fever, nausea, and even vomiting; so that the affection may be mistaken for severe bilious or typhoid fever. In one case, I found the disease had been diagnosed as an inflammatory affection of the brain. An examination of the eye, however, will correct the diagnosis at once. The lids will be found puffy and swollen, the conjunctiva injected, there is chemosis, more or less cloudiness of the aqueous humor, discoloration of the iris, which appears bulged forward almost against the cornea, dilatation of the pupil, and decided tension of the eyeball. Vision is always greatly impaired. I have never known it wholly lost at this stage, although this has not unfrequently happened. Patients will generally see a hand held very near the eye, or be able to distinguish the large gilt letters on the back of a book. They are also disposed to speak of sudden flashes of light before the eyes, and perhaps other spectral phenomena. The above, with some photophobia and lachrymation, are the marked symptoms observed in the beginning of confirmed glaucoma.

As the acute attack passes away, the sight will grow better, and perhaps be almost wholly restored, but the appearance of the eye with a modification of the severe inflammatory aspect, remains. The attacks re-occur, the sight being left after each in a worse condition. The tension of the eye increases, the iris shrivels, the anterior chamber becomes still narrower, the subconjunctival veins become turbid and tortuous, the field of vision becomes very much contracted, the sensibility of the cornea diminished, the so-called green reflex is marked. I say so-called green reflex, because I find the green usually absent. The reflex, to my eye, is simply slate-colored. No doubt it is sometimes *greenish*. The peculiar hue is produced in the glaucomatous eye of an elderly person by admixture or blending of the reflex from a brownish-yellow lens, with a dirty bluish-gray aqueous humor. The result is a very dirty greenish reflex, which to me is scarcely green at all. There is sometimes a bluish-green to be seen, but if one looks for a decided green reflex, such as is frequently noticed in the eye of a cat, he will be disappointed. The diminished sensibility of the cornea is easily determined by touching it with a bit of paper twisted to a point.

THE OPHTHALMOSCOPIC SYMPTOMS,

In the premonitory stage, are wholly absent, or at most, frequently of merely negative value, from cloudiness of the aqueous humor. In the stage of confirmed glaucoma, there may be more or less excavation of the optic disc, dilation, and turgescence and tortuosity of the retinal veins, and venous pulsation. At a later stage of the disease we may find the arteries thin and pale, arterial pulsation, hemorrhage into and general cloudiness of the vitreous. The large excavation of the optic nerve differs from the physiological and amaurotic excavations, in size, depth, and in the abruptness of its edge, in consequence of which the retinal vessels, in curling over the margin at the border of the disc, are much displaced. Frequently, however, the media in glaucoma are so turbid that nothing whatever can be seen with the ophthalmoscope. Fortunately, when this is the case, the other symptoms are so characteristic that no error in diagnosis need occur.

Sub-acute glaucoma does not differ in character from the acute. The symptoms are less severe, and its course less rapid, but the end is similar. It is not necessary to describe it.

Chronic inflammatory glaucoma is merely an advanced stage of the acute form when the exacerbations having diminished somewhat in intensity, the inflammation is fixed and gradually progressive, and the sight gradually failing.

Chronic non-inflammatory glaucoma, sometimes called glaucoma simplex, is very insidious in its course, and of rare occurrence compared to other forms of the affection. It has not very unfrequently happened that patients have been unaware of the existence of this disease in one eye, the other being well, until it has completely destroyed the sight. Generally the disease is far advanced before aid is sought. Vision fails, glasses are not of service, there may be a slight inflammatory attack, and they seek surgical advice. Frequently the eye appears normal, with perhaps the exception of a slightly dilated and sluggish pupil. That constant and characteristic symptom of glaucoma, increased tension of the globe, is usually present, and the ophthalmoscope will show a glaucomatous excavation of the optic nerve. As the disease progresses, sooner or later inflammatory symptoms are apt to be manifested, as in the inflammatory forms previously spoken of. Whether this be the case or not, the eye gradually assumes the glaucomatous aspect as the globe grows harder.

Glaucoma fulminans is the name given by Professor Graefe to a very rare form of glaucoma, the most dangerous of all, in which the disease progresses with such fearful rapidity, that the sight of a previously sound eye may be wholly destroyed in a few hours, or even in half an hour.

Absolute glaucoma, as the disease is termed, when all perception of light has disappeared, is frequently distinguished at a glance by a pale-greenish opacity of the lens. At this stage of the affection the patient may suffer from severe attacks of ciliary neuralgia. Later, the iris becomes completely atrophied, the cornea opaque and softened, the choroid and retina degenerated, and hemorrhagic effusion takes place within the fundus, staphyloma of the sclerotic, and frequently inflammation and atrophy of the globe follow.

THE NATURE AND CAUSE OF GLAUCOMA

Are not yet fully understood. There is first an affection of the iris, ciliary body, and the choroid, then an increase of the humors of the eye, and increased tension and excavation of the optic nerve; then the cornea, sclerotic, and retina become involved. The fact that the sclerotic in this disease is found rigid and unyielding, is supposed to be of importance; for the disease attacks generally only those of an age above thirty-five or forty, in whom the sclerotic coat has already attained a firmness and rigidity unknown in youth. An interesting and perhaps rational theory, is that which attributes the hyper-secretion of the fluids of the eye to some abnormal irritation of the nerves controlling these secretions, this irritation being reflex from the sympathetic. This hypothesis makes the increase of fluids the essence of the disease, and the consequent tension of the globe the cause of the inflammatory symptoms. The interior tissues of the eye become irritable and inflamed from this mechanical pressure, and finally degenerate from disease and lack of nutrition.

TREATMENT.

In the treatment of glaucoma during its premonitory or very earliest stages, I have no doubt we may do much better than our colleagues of the allopathic school. When we reflect that in a great majority of cases there coexist serious constitutional disturbances, such as gout, rheumatism, functional or other disease of the digestive organs, hemorrhoids; and, in females, that the affection is apt to occur at the period of cessation of menstruation, it seems almost impossible to avoid the conclusion that the affection is primarily extraocular; and that seen at the earliest stage, a careful homœopathic medical treatment, combined with strict hygienic regulations, might prove curative. In estimating the effect of our remedies, we must not overlook the circumstance that, with or without treatment, an acute attack in the earliest stage may repeatedly pass off leaving the sight unimpaired. No doubt our remedies may prove very serviceable in relieving or shortening the duration of an attack, but, to be curative, they must prevent its recurrence, just as the operation of iridectomy when successful prevents its recurrence. In order to afford remedies the best possible chance of proving of permanent benefit, they should be administered also during the period of intermission. We can only be sure that the treatment is proving of real service when we find that *it reduces the hardness of the globe.* Whatever will reduce the tension of the eyeball in glaucoma will cure it. It is probably the intraocular pressure that, long continued, produces blindness.

In addition to the faithful and long-continued administration of remedies, the habits of our patients should be scrupulously looked after. Of course, a most moderate use only of the eyes should be allowed; bright lights and crowded places are to be avoided, sunlight to be modified and deprived of its piercing yellow rays by the use of light blue glasses when in the open air, especially to be used to protect the eyes from the sunlight upon the snow, white sand, or water. In addition to this, all habits which affect the general health unfavorably, such as excessive use of tobacco, alcohol, or other stimulants, all dissipations and exhaustive labor, mental or physical, should be strictly prohibited, under penalty of loss of sight.

The diet should be attended to, any idiosyncrasies of the patient in this respect ferreted out, and indigestible articles forbidden. The diet, however, should be good and nutritious, and, particularly in elderly persons, the confirmed habit of indulgence in stimulants like tobacco, alcohol, tea, and coffee should not be interfered with, unless it be necessary to substitute moderation for excess.

Merc., I believe, to be one of the remedies upon which reliance should be placed in glaucoma. It would seem to be equally indicated whether the complications be of hepatic, hemorrhoidal, or uterine character. Ham., collin., arn., and nux v. will often be useful where hemorrhoidal complications are present. Kali iod. is, in my experience, always useful in inflammations and congestions of the choroid. Arsen., phyto., colch., macrot., spig., and bry. may be serviceable for rheumatic and arthritic symptoms, and, with many other remedies, will be useful when indicated by symptoms apparently only remotely connected with the disease of the eye.

A serious obstacle to the success of the medical treatment of this disease lies in the fact that patients rarely consult a physician until the disease is confirmed, and too great changes have occurred in the fundus to be completely stayed through constitutional means. Many patients sent to me are such as have been completely blind for months, and sometimes years. In other cases of complete blindness, an operation is indicated simply for the relief of a tormenting neuralgia over the eye. No restoration of sight is possible. Only now and then does a case present itself at the most favorable time for a successful operation. If we inquire into the cause of the delay, we find that no attention whatever was paid to the early symptoms; the attack was regarded as a headache, a rheumatism from cold, a neuralgia in the head, or something else of a trivial nature, and no advice was sought until after the advent of a terrible attack of acute inflammation, or until the sight was found permanently impaired, and spectacles of no service.

It is very difficult to relieve the severe ciliary neuralgia which occurs so often in acute attacks, except by surgical interference. An iridectomy, and frequently a simple paracentesis of the anterior chamber, will relieve the pain as if by magic. Division of the ciliary muscle will also relieve the pain, and, like the others, accomplishes its result by removing the intraocular pressure. Warm fomentations of simple water or warm water medicated with bell., cham., or opium, are usually of some service. Internally, I have administered mostly bell., spig., cham., con., macrot., merc., and val. of zinc during the paroxysms of severe suffering.

SURGICAL TREATMENT.

Iridectomy in the early stages of glaucoma is almost a certain cure for it. In the later stages, it is always a palliative, and sometimes a cure. The operation is painful, and usually performed under the influence of an anæsthetic. It is similar to the operation for artificial pupil already described, *except that we enter the eye from the sclerotic* near its junction with the cornea, and the opening is as large as the keratome or iridectomy lance will allow. The large opening and the placing it in the sclera, are for the purpose of excising a large segment of the iris, and insuring the section to reach quite back to the ciliary border. This has been demonstrated to insure a more certain and permanent relief of the intraocular pressure. A smaller iridectomy made through the cornea, as in artificial pupil, is not productive of permanent results. After the operation the eye is simply bandaged, and the patient kept quiet for a few days, until the corneal wound heals and the artificially produced irritation is gone. Very rarely is the reaction sufficient to call for the application of cold compresses. The administration of aconite, for a day or two, is always advisable after the operation.

WHEN TO MAKE THE IRIDECTOMY.

An important point to be determined is the length of time we may wait in case our remedies fail of the desired effect before resorting to an operation. The ready answer, and the true answer, to a question of this kind is, *the sooner the operation is performed in a case of glaucoma* the better. Delays are exceedingly dangerous. But the patient is not often willing at the very commencement of the disease to submit to an iridectomy, even if we happen to be fortunate enough to be consulted thus early. As a rule, then, he may safely postpone the operation so long as the intermissions of congestion, pain, and blindness *are complete*. When there is simply *re*mission instead of *inter*mission the eye is in great danger, and if vision is continuously impaired, and especially if *the field of vision is contracted*, the operation should be postponed no longer than is absolutely necessary. We must, as before observed, always bear in mind that with or without medical treatment the subjective symptoms are constantly changing, and that, while our measures may be palliative, they cannot be curative unless they reduce the abnormal tension (hardness) of the globe. In the estimation of this tension we are to be guided by our sense of touch, rather than by any sensations of the patient. Both his eyes being closed, we press very gently, either together or in alternation, upon both eyeballs, determining their comparative hardness, and comparing them in this respect, if necessary, with our own.

The prognosis, when iridectomy is performed in the premonitory or the very early stage of acute inflammatory glaucoma, is favorable. Tension is reduced, vision perfectly recovered, and the eye restored to a healthy condition. In order that this success should be nearly certain, the patient should, before operating, be still able to see large print, and the disease in its confirmed state ought not to be of more than a week or two in duration. Still, success may crown an operation in acute glaucoma when vision is reduced to a mere perception of light, and good sight be permanently restored.

In later stages of acute glaucoma, if vision be not too much impaired, and the field of vision not much contracted, permanent good results may be looked for; but if the reverse of this obtains, the visual field is narrow, sight very much impaired, and the excavation of the optic nerve considerable, the result of the operation, though good, and offering the only chance for the patient, may not be permanent.

In subacute and chronic glaucoma we may expect to prevent further loss of vision and preserve the eye from future inroads of the disease, provided sight is not wholly gone and the field of vision is not too much narrowed. In these cases, indeed, vision sometimes improves considerably; not rapidly always, as after an operation in acute glaucoma, but after the lapse of some months. In non-inflammatory glaucoma the prognosis is not quite so favorable, unless the operation be performed while there is still considerable vision left. In glaucoma fulminans, performed early, the operation has been successful.

In absolute glaucoma, when all perception of light is gone, the operation of iridectomy is only indicated to cure pain, and prevent the recurrence of the inflammatory attacks. According to my own experience, it is almost certain to do this.

It is not surprising when we consider that the operation of iridectomy offers a chance, however slight it may be, of restoring sight even in old and unfavorable cases, that it should often be performed against all indications, and even against all hope, and as a natural consequence that it should often fail. This occasions disappointment, and sometimes distrust of the value of the operation generally. It must not be forgotten, however, that there are pretty definite indications in the state of the patient's vision which cannot be ignored, if we wish our prognosis to prove correct, and that it is rather too much to expect of any operation that it shall prove successful when not indicated. It is not affirmed of the operation that it is a sure cure for glaucoma, but simply that *when indicated* it is the only reliable cure for glaucoma known at the present time, and that in a vast majority of instances it has proved successful.

The rationale of iridectomy in this disease is not demonstrated as yet. The theories advanced on this point are neither remarkable nor attractive enough to make it worth while to devote sufficient of our limited space to their examination. We know that iridectomy at its best permanently reduces tension, but *how* it does this is still a question.

OTHER OPERATIONS FOR THE CURE OF GLAUCOMA

Are those of division of the ciliary muscle and paracentesis corneæ. The first has not proved as permanent and certain in its results as would be desirable, and the second requires a too frequent repetition to be generally feasible. Both of these procedures are serviceable as has been stated, in temporarily relieving ciliary neuralgia, and may sometimes answer the purpose of relieving pain in those old cases of glaucoma where the sight is irrevocably lost, and nothing more than relief from intolerable suffering is hoped for.

SECONDARY GLAUCOMA.

Glaucoma sometimes supervenes upon injuries of the eye, and more rarely from deep-seated disease of the globe, such as choroiditis or irido-choroiditis, sympathetic ophthalmia, and other affections. It is to be treated surgically, but the chances of success are greatly lessened.

CHAPTER X.

THE RETINA AND OPTIC NERVE.

RETINAL HYPERÆMIA.

A *hyperœmia of the retina* is more readily diagnosed than a similar condition of the choroid. In the active or arterial form there is some photophobia and lachrymation. In the passive or venous form, these are absent. In the first the ophthalmoscope shows a reddened disc from congestion of the capillary vessels upon its surface, and the larger retinal vessels may be somewhat increased in size. It is difficult to determine this, as in florid persons the vessels appear larger and more active than in pale or lymphatic individuals. If one eye only is affected we can, by comparison, make our diagnosis quite certain. In the venous or passive form the retinal veins are dilated, dark, and perhaps tortuous. We notice venous pulsation, or it can readily be produced by pressure on the eyeball.

THE CAUSE AND TREATMENT.

Very often in these cases we find some abnormal state of the refraction or accommodation. I have treated scores of such cases, — and suitable glasses is the remedy. It is caused also by exposure to bright light or very fine work by artificial light, and a radical change of occupation will do much to promote a cure. Very often there will be found disorder of the heart, liver, or uterus as a cause. Cactus I find admirable in retinal congestions, and especially when heart troubles are present. Bell. and macrotin in connection with uterine symptoms. Merc., leptand., bry., sulph., and nux v., when the liver is at fault; and in other conditions I use opium, collinson., or spigel. and conium. Blue or smoke-colored glasses are advisable for out-of-door use, if the photophobia is considerable. When the affection is very severe, complete rest of the eyes should be enjoined.

RETINITIS.

In the serous form of retinitis we notice, with the ophthalmoscope generally, a veiled or hazy appearance of the retina, less marked at the macula lutea, where the normal membrane is always of diminished thickness, and more decided about the optic disc, which is somewhat swollen from œdema, and its outline rather indistinct. The arteries are normal, but the veins look dark and tortuous.

Externally, the eye looks well. Perhaps the pupil may be slightly dilated and sluggish; but, in my experience, this is not usually the case. Nor are there any of those symptoms of irritability of the eye which are so often and erroneously supposed to exist in iritis, such as photophobia, pain, lachrymation, and the phenomena which accompany retinal hyperæsthesia. The causes of this affection do not differ materially from those mentioned under the Affections of the Retina, previously described, and the treatment must be similar in character, but of course more prolonged, and cannot, in many cases, result as successfully. Our prognosis should be more guarded; for, from the beginning, the sight is more impaired. The veil or cloud grows thicker until frequently the patient is almost totally blind. Frequently, if the disease continues many weeks atrophy of the retina may ensue, and the sight be permanently destroyed. The eyes should always be protected by dark-blue glasses, and no use of them whatever for near objects be permitted.

In retinitis exudativa, the deeper-seated or parenchymous form of retinitis, the ophthalmoscopic appearances of the eye are much more striking. The optic disc is reddish-gray, and its outline indistinct and irregular, so that it is almost impossible to find the line of demarcation between it and the retina. The arteries are more or less diminished in size, and the veins swollen and tortuous, and hidden here and there by extensive exudations of a whitish or grayish color, and blood extravasations are seen in various parts of the retina. The above is an ophthalmoscopic picture of a pathological condition in which the inflammatory condition of the retina has produced hypertrophy, stasis, proliferation of cells, colloid or fatty degeneration and sclerosis; of course the ophthalmoscope will not afford so complete a picture as the above in all cases of the kind, but I have observed on more than one occasion appearances almost exactly corresponding to those described. Even in cases nearly like the above, the blood stasis is sometimes relieved, the exudations and extravasations absorbed, and the patient may regain considerable vision to remain permanently. This, however, is by no means the usual course. It more frequently ends in atrophy of the retina and optic nerve. Vision during the progress of the affection is often tolerable until the region of the macula lutea is invaded. *Micropsia* is often noticed; that is, all objects appear smaller than they really are. If you ask the patient to draw a given circle, he invariably draws it smaller than the reality. This is the result of a derangement in the position of the rods and cones of the inflamed retina upon which the image is caught.

THE CAUSE AND TREATMENT.

The cause is frequently a neglected hyperæmic condition of the retina and optic nerve, disease of the heart, of the abdominal viscera, pregnancy, Bright's disease, diabetes, syphilis, or cerebral affections. The treatment should be directed to the removal of the cause when this can be ascertained. When of syphilitic origin, the treatment will be more apt to result favorably than in cerebral or Bright's disease. Merc. should, I think, be relied upon to meet the retinal indications in this form of the affection, and arsen. and zinc for the nephritic variety, using such other remedies temporarily as the state of the patient's health or any special symptoms may require. Hygienic rules should receive the greatest attention, and the eyes *must always be protected from bright light* by the use of colored spectacles. With the wisest treatment in every respect, the result will often prove unsatisfactory.

BRIGHT'S DISEASE OR RETINITIS ALBUMINURICA.

The ophthalmoscopic appearance of the eyes in Bright's disease does not differ very much from that already described, except at a later stage of the affection, when we sometimes find around the optic disc a broad, white ring, and in the region of the macula lutea small stellated white spots, which are later merged in the general exudation.

The pathological changes are principally the serous infiltration of nerve and retina, — the fatty degeneration making the white patches, hypertrophied and sclerosed nerve fibres, giving rise to a striated appearance of the fundus under the ophthalmoscope, capillary hemorrhages, due either to disorder of the circulation from hypertrophy and dilatation of the left ventricle, which is almost always present in Bright's disease, or to disease of the coats of the vessels.

Sight is very much impaired, although the extent of the field of vision is not limited greatly. Certain portions of the field are generally faulty, and of course vision is rarely very acute. Sudden amaurosis is liable to occur in this disease from uræmic poisoning. The patient becomes suddenly blind, and suffers from headache, vertigo, sickness, convulsions, and other general symptoms of uræmic poison.

Why disease of the retina and kidney so uniformly coexist is not known. It has happened not unfrequently that failing sight, and the consequent ophthalmoscopic examination of the fundus of the eye, has led to the detection of disease of the kidney, confirmed by later microscopical examination of the urine. As a rule, nephritic retinitis does not lead to complete loss of sight; but normal vision, in cases of any severity, is not always regained. The amount of vision retained will finally be determined by the extent of disease of the nervous structure of the retina. If this has been great it may lead to atrophy and blindness. The prognosis is, of course, most favorable in albuminuria after fevers or in pregnancy. The treatment, as far as the eye is concerned, will be merely hygienic, and medication must be directed to the cure of the primary seat of the disease, — the kidney.

SYPHILITIC RETINITIS, OR CHOROIDO-RETINITIS,

Does not present so characteristic a picture for the ophthalmoscope, and the history of the case with the constitutional symptoms sometimes require to be consulted before the diagnosis is rendered certain. The appearance of the fundus is striated, and similar to that in retinitis albuminurica, but not so well marked. The stellated spots in the region of the macula lutea appear and disappear rapidly, and the vision improves and retrogrades correspondingly. Extravasations of blood are not usually noticed. *The pathological changes* are serous infiltration of retina, inflammation and degeneration of the choroid, but fortunately the nervous structure of the retina is less apt to be impaired, and our prognosis is therefore favorable, and especially so if the disease comes early under treatment. The disease is usually coincident with the constitutional symptoms of secondary syphilis, and the treatment must be directed to the removal of the constitutional affection. The retinitis progresses very slowly, and the patient is often troubled by relapses. The visual disturbance presents very nearly the same features as in retinitis nephritica. The choroid is usually involved, and the treatment recommended for choroiditis will generally be applicable in this form of retinitis.

IN RETINITIS APOPLECTICA

There is great tendency to extravasations of blood, which are sometimes so extensive as to hide partially the vessels of the retina, and the infiltrations are slighter, and serous in character. The sight is not so much impaired as the ophthalmoscopic appearance of the eye would indicate, unless the hemorrhage is situated about the yellow spot. The disease shows great tendency to relapses, and if hemorrhages recur often, and are at all extensive, our prognosis is not so favorable as otherwise. Apoplexy of the retina is caused by disturbances of the general circulation, frequently due to tumors within the orbit or cranium, which prevent the return of venous blood from the eye. Hypertrophy of the left ventricle or disease of the aortic valves, is not a very unusual cause. In elderly persons, degeneration of the coats of the retinal vessels may be the cause. It would be very difficult to state the precise treatment to be adopted in such cases. The general health should be made as perfect as possible, and the patient should, of course, be scrupulously correct and regular in his habits. Further than this, the general aspect of each case must determine the course to be pursued in regard to medicine, diet, change of air, climate, and the like.

RETINITIS PIGMENTOSA,

As its name indicates, is an inflammation of the retina characterized chiefly by great pigmentation. The ophthalmoscope reveals the disease at a glance. The retina is covered by large irregular patches of pigment, more at the periphery of the fundus where the deposit commences first. The veins are enlarged, the arteries diminished in calibre, the choroid becomes degenerated, so that its vessels are visible, and even the glistening sclera may often be seen shining through it. In such a case the fundus presents a wonderfully mottled and parti-colored picture under the ophthalmoscope.

The striking subjective symptom in this affection is night blindness. This is the result of a torpid condition of the retina, produced by the insufficient supply of blood through the narrowed vessels, in consequence of which the retina requires a bright light to receive the impression of objects. This disease must not be confounded with a functional disorder of the retina called hemeralopia, or night blindness, mentioned under Amblyopia. The field of vision is often very much diminished in extent, so that while in a direct line one may still read fine print, all around may be involved in darkness.* The disease is generally congenital, or hereditary, and sooner or later leads to blindness. It often occurs in marriages of consanguinity and with deaf-mutism. Treatment can only be palliative, but this may undoubtedly postpone blindness for years. The patient's general health should be kept in the best possible condition, and above all, the eyes should be spared fatiguing occupations, and guarded from bright light and heat.

DETACHMENT OF THE RETINA

Is occasioned by serous effusion between it and the choroid. It most frequently occurs in the lower half of the fundus, and commences at the periphery. With the ophthalmoscope we must look for it always by *direct examination*. The light need not be very

---

* In a patient of mine, a student of Harvard College, the extent of the field of vision is so limited at the distance of one foot, that its size is just about realized with a normal eye, in looking through a tube eight inches in length and a half inch in diameter.

strong. Notice that the bright red of the fundus is only seen at the upper part of the pupil; all below is dark; or perhaps you catch the illuminated part of the pupil only after directing the patient to turn his eye in different directions. Do not approach the eye too nearly, and you will see by carefully regarding the un-illuminated part of the pupil, and apparently almost in contact with it, a grayish blue cloud which undulates with every movement of the eye. For lack of the simple precaution of using the *upright image*, and regarding the eye from the distance of twelve or fifteen inches at first, I have known an excellent ophthalmoscopist to overlook a large detachment of the retina. Once having made the diagnosis, we may examine the details with either the direct or reversed image. We find the floating opacity or retinal cloud crossed by dark, shrivelled, crooked vessels. Slight degrees of detachment of the retina are much more difficult to diagnose. This is sometimes best accomplished by commencing with a retinal vessel at the optic disc and following it towards the periphery, where we may detect a change to a darker color, and a tortuousness in its course; and we make out at the same time a slight fold in the retina.

Vision is, as a matter of course, very much impaired. That portion of the retina separated from the choroid by serous effusion, no longer performs its function; but the part which maintains its connection with the choroid performs its function as usual. Hence it happens that the upper part of the field of vision is entirely obscured, or, if the detachment happen to have occurred in the upper part of the fundus, the obscurity is in the lower part of the visual field. Impaired vision is first noticed by the patient as a delicate cloud with indistinct wavy outline, at that point in the field of vision corresponding exactly to the situation of the effusion beneath the retina in the fundus. Linear objects appear wavy and broken, due, probably, to the disturbed connection of the retina at the edge of the detachment.

The cause of the disease is sometimes difficult to determine. It is frequently occasioned by a blow on the eye. In a patient of mine, during the past year, it could be traced directly to a fall a few months previous. It is due, not unfrequently, to hemorrhage in disease of the choroid or retina. The commonest cause is, perhaps, the elongation of the optic axis, as seen in myopic patients. The choroid adheres to the sclera, and is distended with it; but as the less elastic retina is not, its connection with the choroid becomes weakened, and any effusion finds its way easily beneath it.

The prognosis is unfavorable, as the separation generally goes on until the eye is rendered blind.

Fortunately it is, in a vast majority of instances, confined to one eye. Sometimes, however, the disease ceases to progress after reaching a certain point, and the sight may improve; and if the detachment is not too extensive, sight may be wholly restored through the absorption of the exudation and reunion of the retina and choroid. I have no doubt that, under favorable conditions for proper medical and hygienic treatment, this result might often be reached. I have had no opportunity of testing the effects of judicious treatment: of the five cases which I have had in private practice, three were old and incurable, and the others lived too far away to be under my control. The general health would guide us chiefly in the selection of internal remedies, but I have no doubt that merc., ars., hepar, kali iod., and some other of our remedies, might exercise a controlling influence over the affection.

Surgically, the disease is treated by puncture of the retina, allowing the fluid to escape into the vitreous, or to be drawn from the eye. The puncture is made through the sclera at a point corresponding to the detachment, with a sharp needle or with a minute trocar. Temporary improvement usually follows, and sometimes the improvement in vision has been known to continue several months, and, in a few instances, one or two years.

GLIOMA RETINÆ

Is the name given by Virchow to a tumor originating in the retina, and occurring mostly in young children, known generally by the name of encephaloid disease or fungus hæmatodes. In the commencement of the affection, the eye appears healthy externally, and there is no pain. The pupil is, however, more or less dilated, and the sight of the eye is gone. The disease is readily diagnosed with the ophthalmoscope at this stage; a circumscribed portion of the retina is mottled, opaque, and thickened in appearance. Soon the growth protrudes as a yellowish-white mass into the vitreous humor, and its vascular character in all its detail is observable. Rapidly now the growth increases, pushing before it the lens and iris, augmenting the intraocular pressure and pain, the cornea or anterior portion of the sclera bursts, and the tumor increases still more rapidly. It assumes later a dark hue from exposure to the atmosphere, exudes a sanious fluid which becomes incrusted on its surface, and bleeds easily.

The prognosis is always grave, and especially so if the disease is in an advanced stage. If the patient is seen early, the eye should be immediately enucleated, as cases are recorded where, after the lapse of several years, the disease has not returned. The optic nerve, in performing the operation, should be excised far back near the optic foramen, so as to include the whole of the diseased portion, if possible. Even after the tumor has burst through the eye an operation will give the only chance of prolonging life, and will certainly alleviate a great amount of suffering. The tumor breaks through, and appears externally in from one to three years from its commencement.

The cause of glioma is often very obscure. It occurs most frequently in children from two to ten years old. It is sometimes complicated with cerebral disease, as evidenced by headache, drowsiness, stupor, or paralytic symptoms. It is often hereditary. I have seen two of four children of the same mother affected by it.

Ischæmia retinæ is a name given to an extremely anæmic condition of the retina, which has been noticed a few times, and has been cured by removing the intraocular pressure by paracentesis of the cornea or by an iridectomy.

Complete paralysis of the retina and total blindness have been observed after blows, and after a stroke of lightning. The ophthalmoscope does not always reveal the great change which one might expect to find under such circumstances.

Embolism of the central artery of the retina is a

rare disease. I have noticed the publication of only one case in this country. The loss of sight in these cases is sudden, and almost total. The ophthalmoscope shows a pale optic disc, transparent however, and the vessels running over it much attenuated. The arteries of the retina are very small, and partially bloodless, so that at certain points of their course they appear like white threads. The veins of the retina present a somewhat similar appearance, though less strongly marked. Later, a bluish opacity is observable in the region of the macula lutea. The disease is sometimes, but not uniformly, accompanied by valvular disease of the heart. Probably the class of remedies indicated in cardiac affections might frequently be of service in this disease. Patients recover, in exceptional cases, sufficient sight to be able to read with the affected eye.

OPTIC-NEURITIS.

Optic-neuritis, or *neuro-retinitis*, is the name given to a condition in which the optic nerve is the primary seat of the inflammation. This condition is very often connected with disease of the brain. Vision is generally greatly impaired, and in a large number of instances, atrophy of the retina and optic nerve and blindness ensue. This sad termination, however, is not always certain. Even when the affection is cerebral in origin the sight may remain unimpaired. A good prognostic symptom is afforded by testing the extent of the field of vision. If this is diminished in extent we may expect more or less atrophy of the nerve. When the affection comes from the brain, there will usually be cerebral symptoms preceding, such as headache, giddiness, vomiting, failure of memory, loss of taste, hearing, smell, convulsive or paralytic attacks. In all cerebral fevers optic-neuritis should be looked for with the ophthalmoscope, because it may exist for some time before vision is sufficiently impaired to direct our attention to the eye. In all suspected disease of the brain, of whatever nature, the ophthalmoscope should also be resorted to as an aid to diagnosis.

The ophthalmoscopic symptoms in the beginning are a hyperæmia and œdema of the disc, which is reddish, its outline indistinct, and afterwards quite indefinable, loss of its transparency, while the effusion of lymph in the optic nerve gives it a striated and woolly aspect. The inflammation extends to the retina, rendering it hazy, its veins dark and tortuous, its arteries shrunken so as hardly to be visible, the vessels here and there hidden in their course beneath the infiltration. Around the disc are blood extravasations, and the exudations upon the disc itself are sometimes so considerable that the vessels upon it are completely covered, and can only be traced to its margin, followed from the retina. Although both nerve and retina are usually involved, when the origin of the affection is cerebral, it is more limited to the optic nerve, — a *neuritis* rather than a *neuro-retinitis*.

The disease does not always, fortunately, present so unfavorable an aspect as this. In young and delicate females, for instance, it is much less grave usually, and the prognosis, when they come early under care, is more favorable. These cases are not cerebral, and indeed the patients are sometimes otherwise in good health. Generally, however, there is catamenial disorder, more or less spinal irritation, and abnormal sensibility of the central nervous system. In a case of this kind under my care two years since, that of a young girl of seventeen, from New Hampshire, there were no catamenial troubles, but considerable spinal irritation in the region of the lower cervical vertebræ. She suffered also from congestive headaches in the forehead and temporal region, general irritability with perhaps slight attacks of hysteria. She was perfectly healthy looking, well formed, but not very robust. When she came to me vision was very imperfect. Jan. 5, 1867, she reads No. 8 print with the right eye and only No. 13 with the left. There is hyperæmia of the optic disc in both eyes, and in the left fundus, the disc and its immediate vicinity are slightly obscured by a delicate reddish-gray haze. The pupils are abnormally dilated, but not much sluggishness is observable in their response to the action of light. Field of vision nearly normal in extent. Photophobia not marked, and no pain in the eyes. Bell. and merc., in alternation, were prescribed. Jan. 24. — Patient about the same in general health. Sight of right eye the same; of the left, a little worse. Acuteness of vision with the best eye about one-eighth; that is, print that a normal eye could read at twenty-four feet she could only read at three feet. Partly owing to her obstinate attacks of congestive headache, I prescribed cactus and sanguin. in alternation night and morning. March 6. — Her headaches are less frequent and violent, and her sight in the right eye has improved. Acuteness of vision about one-quarter. The left eye is no worse: continued medicine. March 27. — Better: acuteness of vision three quarters. Left eye better. May 17. — She can read No. 1 test type with either eye. General health very much improved. The cause of the disease in this case was very obscure. Fortunately the affection in the left eye did not progress so far as to occasion any structural alterations in the nervous element of the retina. A rather curious feature of the case remains to be stated. More than seven months after she passed from under my observation she called on me, stating that her eyes had remained well, but that she believed she was getting near-sighted. On examination I found a myopia of about one-twelfth, for which concave glasses, of fourteen-inch focus, were prescribed. It would seem that this myopia should be the result of a sclerotico-choroiditis posterior, but I saw no ophthalmoscopic indications of the existence of this affection. Eleven months later, on Dec. 3, 1868, my patient visited me again to see if I thought her glasses the proper ones for her to wear. She had recently begun to find some fatigue of the eye in wearing them. I found her myopia less, and substituted glasses of twenty-four inch focus.

In most cases of neuro-retinitis, however, the prognosis should be very guarded. It will be most favorable, of course, when the affection can be traced to disorder of the uterine or some other important function that admits of a cure, and also in cases that supervene on convalescence from febrile disorders, especially if in these instances the ophthalmoscope does not show great or dangerous change of appearance in the optic nerve or retina. *Neuritis descendens* as it is sometimes called, when it arises from intra-cranial causes, generally terminates sooner or later in total blindness. Generally speaking, it has been noticed that when the progress of the disease and loss of sight have been rapid, the prognosis is more favorable than when the progress and loss of sight have been gradual. In relation to the medical treatment, it must of course vary according to the cause, the general health of the patient, and the exigencies of each individual case. Other things being equal, I should trust sooner to merc., ars., zinc, aurum, kali iod., and phosph., than to bell., nux, cactus, gelsem., con., spig., macrot, and crocus, although the last mentioned will, some of them, be called for as intercurrents in many cases.

ATROPHY OF THE OPTIC NERVE,

Amaurosis, *cerebral or cerebro-spinal amaurosis*. I limit the signification of the term amaurosis to primary disease or degeneration of the optic nerve. (See chapter on Amblyopia.) A marked symptom of amaurosis, noticeable at a glance, is the dilated and sluggish pupil, and generally, when the eye is quite blind, its complete immobility. Exceptionally the pupil retains its activity, and, in spinal amaurosis, it may even be contracted.

The ophthalmoscopic appearances of the fundus are very characteristic. The nerve disc is pale, from the attenuation or disappearance of the small nutrient vessels on its face, there is bluish or bluish-green discoloration, especially seen in spinal amaurosis, the transparency of the disc is lost, its outline is clear and distinct, the retinal vessels are generally diminished in size, notably the arteries, and there is frequently an excavation of the optic nerve. This excavation must be distinguished from a very slight physiological one, which is congenital and often seen in the normal eye, situated at the centre or a little towards the temporal side of the disc. In the physiological excavation of course none of the symptoms of atrophy above mentioned obtain, the nerve being in its normal condition. In the atrophic excavation, which is shallow, its edges are gradually sloped, quite unlike the abrupt margin of the glaucomatous excavation described under Glaucoma. Hence the retinal vessels, in passing into the cavity from the normal surface of the disc, do not appear under the ophthalmoscope as if displaced, as in glaucoma, but describe simply a curve. Sometimes in the physiological excavation this curve may also be abrupt enough to give a vessel the appearance of displacement.

The patient's sight is more or less impaired, and the field of vision contracted. The proper investigation of the extent and nature of the limitation of the field of vision is of the utmost importance in this affection as determining our prognosis. The contraction of the visual field usually commences at the temporal side, but in glaucoma, at the nasal side.

The contraction of the field may be symmetrical in both eyes, or it may be equilateral; that is, at the temporal half of one and the nasal half of the other. The former is very unfavorable, the latter sometimes a very favorable, symptom. It must be remembered that the optic nerve fibres decussate at the optic commissure, so that the right nerve passes partly to the temporal or right side of the retina of the right eye, and to the nasal or right side of the retina of the left eye, while the left optic nerve supplies the left half of the two retinæ in a corresponding manner. Now, if the temporal side of each field of vision is limited the disease must be seated at the commissure, and this augurs a bad termination. Blindness often comes on very rapidly. But if the field of vision is contracted equilaterally, total blindness is pretty certain not to ensue, indeed rarely or never ensues, unless the disease extend afterwards to the commissure or some new cerebral symptoms manifest themselves.

The patient is also apt to be troubled with dark spots before the eyes. If such a scotoma happen to be seated directly in the axis of vision it proves quite troublesome to sight.

THE CAUSE OF AMAUROSIS

Is sometimes very obscure. Meningitis of the base of the brain is a frequent one, especially in its chronic form, as is also periostitis at the base of the brain. Tumors of the brain, through implication of, or pressure upon, the optic nerve cause progressive atrophy. Disease of the spinal cord may produce the same through the medium of the sympathetic.

Atrophy of the nerve presenting ophthalmoscopic appearances characteristic enough to warrant the name of *tobacco amaurosis*, has been thought by some to exist; but it is by no means proved as yet to differ sufficiently from atrophy due to the excessive use of alcohol, and other enervating habits, to warrant its name. The absorption of lead into the system has been known to produce atrophy of the optic nerve, but consecutive upon neuritis-optica.

THE PROGNOSIS

In atrophy of the optic nerve is bad enough; but, as has been observed, the condition of the field of vision frequently holds out hopes of a not too unfavorable termination. Sudden accession of blindness is not to be considered an unfavorable symptom, especially in children. It is favorable if the disease remains stationary for a considerable time, and bad if it manifest a slow, but certain progress. If the visual field is not contracted after the affection has continued for some time it is a favorable sign, as is likewise the fact of the line of demarcation between the good and bad of the field, being very distinct. Irregular contractions of the visual field occurring simultaneously or in quick succession in both eyes are unfavorable. Central scotoma are unfavorable if the visual field is much contracted, otherwise not particularly so. When the field of vision beyond the scotoma is impaired it shows a lack of the power of transmission on the part of the retina, and progressive atrophy is to be feared. All auxiliary or accompanying symptoms are of great importance, because it is quite impossible to decide from the appearance of the optic nerve alone, whether in many cases the atrophy be progressive or stationary. The medical treatment must differ so much in different cases that I do not know that I can do more than refer the reader to the indications and remarks in regard to treatment made under the head of Neuritis-optica.

CHAPTER XI.

AMBLYOPIC AND OTHER AFFECTIONS.

AMBLYOPIA.

THIS term, strictly speaking, is limited to those cases of imperfect vision in which the affected eye presents no recognizable objective symptoms, with or without the ophthalmoscope, and in which the impaired vision is not due to anomalous refraction, as in hypermetropia, myopia, and astigmatism.

In a general way, the term amblyopia is used to express impaired sight from any and every cause except that of optical defect. Thus we say, if we find that no glasses improve the acuteness of vision, that the patient is amblyopic, — meaning by the remark nothing more definite than that the blindness is not to be attributed wholly to abnormal refractive power, and that some disease of the fundus of the globe is present.

DIAGNOSIS OF AMBLYOPIA.

A simple, practical, and quite reliable method of diagnosing amblyopia, as well as other diseases of the eye, involving loss of vision, from those of anomalous refractive power, requiring only proper glasses for their cure, is by the easy device of permitting the patient to look through a large pinhole in a blackened card. *If this improves vision*, refraction is faulty, and will be corrected by suitable glasses. If vision *is not improved*, the loss of visual power must be sought in some of the inner structures of the eye, and an ophthalmoscopic examination will be necessary. Of course nicer methods than this to determine faulty refraction, when the requisite concave and convex glasses are at hand, are those mentioned in the chapter on Anomalies of Refraction ; but the requisite glasses are frequently not at hand in the office of the general practitioner, and the above test of Giraud Teulon will prove very convenient.

In the January number of the "American Journal of Medical Sciences," Dr. Thomson shows how this test may be made to indicate the exact nature of a case of anomalous refraction. In looking through the pinhole at a gas-light at twenty feet distance, if the eye is ametropic (of defective refractive power), when the card is moved rapidly before the eye, the light will seem to dance. If the eye is emmetropic, the light will remain steady. In testing the eye of a patient in this way I found that the dancing of the light was removed by permitting him to look through

No. 16 concave glasses, — those appeared to render his eye emmetropic. His eye was myopic $\frac{1}{16}$. In another instance the light danced when the card was moved up and down, but not when it was moved horizontally. This indicated ametropia in the vertical meridian, and it was found by trial that a concave cylindrical glass, No 36, the axis horizontal, remedied the defect. The case was one of simple astigmatism. With two pinholes, one-eighth of an inch apart in the card, an emmetropic eye will see one light, an ametropic eye, two. In myopia, the second image will be at the right, in hypermetropia, at the left. In the case of the myope just mentioned, by covering one of the pinholes with a red glass he saw the red flame about eight inches at the right of the yellow, at a distance of forty feet. Through his No. 16 concave glass the red and yellow flames were one. In the case of astigmatism mentioned above, with the two holes held one above the other, at a distance of forty feet, he saw the red flame about four inches above the yellow. His cylindrical glass nearly fused the two images. In determining a hypermetropia by this method it will frequently be necessary to first paralyze the accommodation with a solution of atropine. An emmetropic eye may easily be made to test the correctness of these various methods by placing before it a convex glass which renders it myopic, or a concave glass when it becomes hypermetropic, or a cylindrical glass which renders it astigmatic.

CAUSE AND TREATMENT OF AMBLYOPIA.

Temporary congestion of the brain and nervous structure of the eye may be occasioned by suppression of exhalations from the skin through exposure to the cold or wet, by suspension of the catamenia, and by large doses of quinine or other drugs, the result of the congestion being dimness or entire suspension of vision. The reverse of this, a diminished supply of pure blood to the brain and retina, will also produce amblyopia. This enfeebled condition may be due to severe illness, excessive drain on the system through hemorrhage, discharge from the uterus, gestation, too long suckling, and like debilitating causes.

In such instances of impaired vision we should not neglect an ophthalmoscopic examination. Our prognosis will be uncertain unless we can first establish a correct diagnosis. This cannot always be done, but it can often be done. The fact that the ophthalmoscopic examination frequently yields but negative results is of itself a favorable omen for the prognosis. Sometimes the examination of the interior of the eye reveals enough to make the future of the patient extremely doubtful. A few days since a case of amblyopia from pregnancy at the eighth month, was sent to me, and on examination I found an optic neuritis with considerable effusion in the retina. The prognosis needs to be extremely guarded in such instances. Less perceptible changes than this in the fundus of the globe are followed by permanent impairment of vision. A number of cases have been published in which the blindness of pregnancy has terminated unfavorably. The significance of the different limitations of the field of vision is noticed under Atrophy of the Optic Nerve.

We have many remedies suitable for congestion to the nervous tunic of the eye. Cactus I have often given with favorable results in hyperæmia of the retina. Bell. and macrot. I have also given frequently, and less often puls., bry., sang., phosph., glon. and opium. Generally these remedies have been administered with reference to the cause and to the totality of symptoms, including those of the eye. For instance, in menstrual suppression, puls.; in rheumatic cases, bry.; complication of heart troubles, glon., cactus; severe throbbing headache, sang.; rush of blood to the head and epistaxis, phosph. Hot pediluvia are sometimes serviceable, and the judicious use of the Turkish bath will benefit disordered function of the skin. That the Turkish bath will also diminish the flow of blood to the brain has been proved by ophthalmoscopic examination made before and after the bath.

In those cases clearly due to impoverished state of the blood, chin., ferr., arsen., phosph., and other remedies will be indicated; but in addition to the appropriate medicines, a nutritious diet and sufficient rest and sleep should be prescribed. Hemorrhage and all unusual drains on the vitality of the patient must be controlled before improvement can be looked for.

Amblyopia from fright or mental shock might undoubtedly be treated successfully by remedies such as ignat., coff., hyos., or the new ones, cyp., scut., and others.

Blood poisoning, from drugs like lead, and narcotics like alcohol and tobacco, will produce amblyopia. Total abstinence from alcohol and tobacco would seem to be the only course for such as cannot draw the line between a stimulating and narcotizing use of these substances. Drug poisoning requires a specific line of treatment for each case; lead poisoning is said, recently, to be successfully treated by opium, through the hypodermic injection of morphia. Amaurosis may be the direct result of blood poisoning, but even in blanching and apparent atrophy of the optic nerve, a very grave symptom indeed, there are many cases recorded in which a more or less perfect recovery of vision is known to have taken place after the lapse of months or years of blindness.*

Dental neuralgia sometimes impairs vision, through reflex irritation from a branch of the fifth nerve. Removal of the offending tooth generally cures.

The exclusion of an eye from participation in vision is a very common cause of unilateral amblyopia. Of several hundreds of cases of strabismus in which I have tested the acuteness of vision or seen it tested by others, I recall few in which a certain degree of monocular amblyopia was not present. This subject is discussed more fully under the head of Strabismus. The cure for amblyopia produced in this way is, in exercising the eye regularly, either with or without a convex glass, according to the degree of vision still left it. The eyes of children become amblyopic much sooner when excluded from participation in sight than those of adults.

Temporary, and indeed persistent, amblyopia is sometimes due to disorders of digestion from impaired functional or other disease of the stomach or liver. These affections cause, through the medium of the sympathetic nerve, some disturbance in the nervous structure of the eye whereby vision is impaired. The

* *Vide* "Royal London Ophthalmic Hospital Reports," Vol. VI., Part iii.

same effect is produced on the sight, occasionally, from nervous or other apparently slight affections of the uterus. In these instances, especially if the ophthalmoscope shows no changes in the interior of the eye sufficiently marked to account for the visual disturbance, the treatment must be directed chiefly to the cure of the disordered viscera.

SIMULATION OF BLINDNESS

In one eye, by nervous or hysterical persons, by conscripts or prisoners, is readily detected by holding the finger or a ruler midway between the eyes and the print while the patient reads. If the patient sees with only one eye, vision will be interrupted, if with both, not. If this is not wholly satisfactory, by moving the ruler slightly from side to side so as to cover each eye in alternation, any further simulation of blindness will generally be detected. The deception may also be shown by means of a prism, base inwards or outwards, before the normal eye. If there is a corrective squint or change in the direction of the eyes as the prism is removed, binocular vision is proved, or the base of the prism being upward or downward, if the patient sees double, binocular vision is certain. The stereoscope may also be used as a test, as binocular vision is requisite in order to appreciate its effects. Simulation of blindness *in both eyes*, may be detected by observing the action of light on the size of the pupil. Mobility of the iris under the stimulus of light is a tolerably sure indication of sight in one or both eyes.

HEMERALOPIA, OR NIGHT BLINDNESS,

Is generally considered a purely functional disease of the retina, in which no changes are observable with the ophthalmoscope. It is an affection confined in its origin almost wholly to warm climates, and will be remembered as one from which our soldiers on duty in the extreme South suffered considerably. Sailors, in tropical regions, are also frequent sufferers. The distinguishing characteristic of the disease is, a torpor of the retina, so that a bright light is required in order to stimulate it sufficiently to receive distinct impressions of objects; hence by night the patient's sight is unusually bad. The time of the day has no significance, such as the name of the affection would indicate; for by a bright artificial light, he sees as well by night as if no affection of the eye were present.

The cause of the disease is exposure to glare of light, and impoverished condition of the blood. Both these conditions are present with our soldiers and sailors in warm latitudes. It is often met with in conjunction with malarial fevers, and the ill-fed and ill-housed peasants in the south of Europe and in Central America are subject to it. Sailors afflicted with scurvy are often subjects of it.

The treatment is very simple and efficacious. Rest, protection of the eyes from bright light, such constitutional remedies as are necessary for the restoration of the general health, or change of climate, generally cure speedily. In Italy, where the affection is quite common, a popular remedy among the people is fumigation with the vapor from the liver of a sheep or other animal. Quaglino, and some others, have observed symptoms of retinitis in the ophthalmoscopic appearance of the fundus of the eye in this affection. Night blindness is a prominent symptom also of the disease called retinitis pigmentosa. In this affection the field of vision becomes limited, a subjective symptom which is characteristic enough to distinguish it clearly from hemeralopia.

COLOR BLINDNESS

Is sometimes congenital. In these cases there is usually an inability to distinguish the shades of red, and red from its complementary color, green. *Achromatopsia*, inability to distinguish all colors, is due to disease of the optic nerve or optic nerve and retina. It has been noticed also as a symptom of myelitis.

HYPERÆSTHESIA RETINÆ, OR RETINAL ASTHENOPIA,

Is characterized by severe photophobia, lachrymation, and all the symptoms of an irritation of the ciliary plexus of nerves. There are no ophthalmoscopic changes observable in the fundus of the globe. In cases which have come under my care there has been, uniformly, dilatation of the pupil. The sight is good in a diminished light, but the field of vision is usually somewhat contracted. It occurs mostly in young females in delicate health, of irritable nerves, hysterical, and suffering from catamenial disorder. The disease of the nervous structure of the eye is but an indication of the state of the nervous system generally, and the treatment must be directed to the removal of the constitutional symptoms. I have found quite a variety of remedies necessary in different cases, and sometimes in the same case. Macrotin, I believe to be more widely serviceable than any other one remedy, but I have frequently given puls., nux, gels., ignat., hyos., scut., bell., and con., according to general indications; gels. is not as reliable in photophobia perhaps as many remedies, but I do not find this symptom to contraindicate it. Blue glasses should be worn in the open air, and it may be necessary to moderate the light to a certain extent in-doors. I have never yet found it necessary to confine persons for days in complete darkness, as has been practised and recommended. Indeed, it has seemed better to encourage the patient in attempting to accustom the eyes gradually to the daylight, as the general health is improved. The strong light is unpleasant rather than injurious. I never hesitate to use the ophthalmoscope freely in these cases, throwing a strong light directly into the eye. No sensitiveness whatever is noticed under the examination after the first few seconds, and I never heard of any after ill effects.

Anæsthesia retinæ is an affection produced by exposure of the eyes to extremely bright light for a long time. *Snow blindness* is a form of this disorder and it is frequently brought on by continued application of the eyes under strong artificial light. The blindness takes the form of a cloud before the eyes, and may be of only short duration, or may continue for weeks. I was the subject of the affection myself during the past summer. After gazing out upon the ocean from a pleasant window for an hour, on going down on to the green lawn I found that the grass appeared to be veiled by an exceedingly delicate blue haze. My friends declared that no such haze existed, and after a few minutes' rest, I saw no more of it. My own case is the only one I have treated, and doubtless the same treatment, rest, and perhaps some safeguard against a too bright light, will generally effect a restoration of acute vision.

NEURALGIA OCULI

Is usually associated with, or is merely a symptom of, a disease of the eye such as iritis, choroiditis, glaucoma, or some other affection, the treatment of which has been already indicated. In hysteria, it is but a phase of the neuralgias common in that disorder of the nervous system, and can only be cured by restoring the general health of the patient. It may be relieved by such measures as are recommended for ciliary neuralgia.

CHAPTER XII.

THE CRYSTALLINE LENS.

CATARACT.

CATARACT is an opacity of the lens, its capsule, or both lens and capsule, and may therefore be called *lenticular*, *capsular*, or *capsulo lenticular*.

DIAGNOSIS.

The subjective symptoms are dimness of vision, in proportion to the age or density of the opacity, which increases gradually, except in traumatic cataract, when it may be sudden, and in congenital cataract. The patient sees better generally in a dim light, because, the pupil being larger, the periphery of the lens is uncovered, and this portion of the lens is usually clearer than the centre. For the same reason the instillation of atropine improves vision somewhat. The first symptom usually noticed by the patient with beginning cataract, is, that distant objects appear slightly hazy, or as if surrounded by a halo; afterwards, as the cataract develops, vision for near objects is similarly impaired.

Objective symptoms. The pupil is generally normal in size and movement. The vacant look, rolling of the eyes, and tendency to look upward of amaurosis is not present. The patient is inclined to look downward, and is able usually to fix the eyes on objects. If the affection has made considerable progress, a gray opacity is at once noticed *exactly* filling the area of the pupil, the opacity being sharply limited by the pupillary margin. A corneal opacity may hide a portion of the iris, but a lenticular opacity can only obscure the pupil. The pupil should be enlarged with atropine, and the eye examined by oblique or lateral illumination.

Examination by lateral illumination enables us to determine the extent and nature of the opacity, whether complete or ripe, its color, its formation, whether nuclear or striated, and other details.

Direct examination with the ophthalmoscope is chiefly serviceable in detecting slight and beginning opacity of the lens, which would otherwise escape observation. The light should not be very strong, and the eye of the observer should be twelve or fifteen inches from that of the patient. There may be a general, but very slight, cloudiness of the whole lens, or the nucleus alone may be obscure, or delicate striæ may be seen running from the periphery towards the centre of the lens. These opacities will appear black instead of grayish, as in the lateral examination. Beginning cataract may be confounded with separation of the retina, a fact which is noticed under Retinal Diseases. In cases where the cataract is dense or far advanced, the ophthalmoscopic signs are negative, as no light can be thrown into the eye.

COMPLICATION, WITH OTHER DISEASES OF THE EYE.

The most common complications are, —

The results of iritis,	Softening of the vitreous humor,
Choroiditis,	Sclerotico-choroiditis posterior,
Separation of the retina,	Amblyopia.

We may determine a complication or its absence, by testing the patient's visual power after the cataract is fully matured. He may be able to distinguish night from day, or the light from a window, and to note a hand before his eyes, even at a distance of three feet, and still we should not be justified in pronouncing the retina sound beyond a doubt. To render the absence of all complications sure, the patient should be able to discern a dim light in a darkened room at a distance of ten to fifteen feet. There should be no contraction of the field of vision as tested by moving a lighted candle from one part of the visual field to the other. The patient's eyes should be fixed on his finger at the distance of a foot during this test, and the candle should be shaded while its position is being changed; the tension of the eyeball should be noticed, and in cases of doubt the whole history of the failure of sight investigated thoroughly. Pain, photophobia, flashes of light, spectra, and like symptoms, are to be regarded as indicating unfavorable complications.

THE CAUSE

Is probably faulty nutrition of the lens. This may be due to old age, as in *senile cataract;* to disease of the kidney, as in *diabetic cataract;* or to abnormal change in the deep structure of the eye, as in *secondary cataract.* There is also a *congenital cataract* dating from birth, and a *traumatic cataract,* from injury. Opacities of the lens fall, practically, into two great divisions, the hard and soft.

HARD OR SENILE CATARACTS

Are distinguished from soft cataracts by their color, which is gray, and approaching the centre, yellowish-gray; they are of uniform appearance, or more frequently striated, the striæ presenting a pearly aspect. Senile cataract is also probable in all opacities of the lens in subjects above the age of fifty. Soft cataracts occur generally in younger persons, and are known by a lighter, more bluish tint, are less apt to be striated, or, if so, the striæ are less symmetrically arranged. Sometimes it is difficult to decide, when the age of the patient furnishes little help, whether a cataract be hard or soft. Less common forms of hard cataract than the *nuclear*, where the nucleus is opaque, the marginal portion remaining for a time transparent, and the *striated* form, presenting lines from the posterior or anterior cortical portion of the lens, or from both, and all running towards the centre, are the so-called *black* cataracts, the centre or nucleus of the lens being dark-brown, and the *siliquose* where the lens is atrophied or over-ripe, and lies in its shrivelled capsule.

The progress of hard cataracts is very variable, sometimes slow for a time, and then rapid. It is better not to answer the invariable question of patients decidedly, as to the time when the cataract will be perfect. It is very certain that a cataract of one eye will, sooner or later, be followed by the same affection in the other.

THE OPERATION OF EXTRACTION

Is indicated as soon as the cataract has ripened. We may judge of this by the appearance of the opacity, which is denser, deeper in color, and extends through the entire lens, so that the shadow of the iris at the circumference of the lens is scarcely visible. The vision is also more indistinct. Dilation of the pupil with atropine is less serviceable, as the periphery of the lens is involved in the opacity. When the cataract matures very slowly, it has been recommended to hasten its development by pricking the transparent portions with a fine needle, and keeping the patient in a darkened room for a few days afterward, until the irritation subsides. We may also operate before the cataract is fully ripe. The disadvantage of this, is, that the transparent cortical portion of the lens being softer than the opaque part, may separate from it, and be left to a great extent in the eye, and act afterwards as a foreign body, irritating the iris, and producing disturbance of vision. Operators are not fully in accord as to the necessity of maturity of the cataract before extraction is indicated. It is safer not to operate on both eyes at once.

THE PROGNOSIS.

The prognosis in extraction is very favorable. In uncomplicated cases there are probably not more than three or four per centum of entire failures.

The operations mostly practised for extraction are the *flap*, the *peripheric-linear*, and the *traction* operations. It is advisable to dilate the pupil before operating, with atropine, particularly on account of the effect of the atropine in keeping up the dilatation, after the extraction, thus lessening somewhat the chances of subsequent iritis.

THE FLAP OPERATION.

The patient being in a recumbent position, a practised assistant separates the lids, the operator fixes the eye by pinching up a fold of the conjunctiva with a pair of small forceps. He then enters the cornea, at its outer edge, with a cataract-knife, carries it steadily forward, cutting out either above or below, and making, according to his predetermined intention, either a superior or inferior flap. Allowing the patient now a moment's respite, the eye is again opened, the needle or cystotome introduced, and the capsule of the lens thoroughly lacerated. This being accomplished, the opaque lens, with or without the aid of gentle pressure upon the eye, emerges slowly from between the lips of the wound. Any remains of the soft cortical substance of the lens are then gently removed with a curette or spatula, and the operation is finished.

Exigencies may arise during an operation like this to modify it somewhat. The corneal wound may have been made too small to admit of the passage of the lens. If so, it must be enlarged by cutting with curved scissors, — a proceeding sometimes difficult, the cornea lying directly upon the iris, there being no anterior chamber in consequence of the escape of the aqueous humor. The knife may have entered the cornea too far from its limbus, too near its centre. In this event, it is necessary to cut out in the sclerotica, and the wound will lie towards the inner canthus of the eye. This may render tedious manipulations necessary, after the opening of the capsule, in order to force the lens inward to a point corresponding to the opening of the wound.

Sometimes, after rupturing the capsule, instead of the lens, we have a gush of vitreous humor from the mouth of the wound. In this case, it is necessary to remove the lens immediately from the eye, by means of a curette, or small spoon.

Deep-seated hemorrhage may occur, especially if the complication of glaucoma exist, and in such event the prognosis is bad. Owing to sudden escape of the aqueous humor the iris may be forced against the knife, and wounded, in making the corneal flap. This may render an iridectomy necessary.

The flap operation may be performed with or without the etherization of the patient. I have seen it performed oftener without, but I prefer myself to do it aided by etherization.

PERIPHERIC-LINEAR EXTRACTION.

This operation, of Von Graefe, requires the etherization of the patient, the recumbent position, and the lids to be separated by a stop-speculum. The eye being held in position by delicate forceps in the left hand of the operator, it is entered with a long, narrow knife (instead of the usual Sichel or Beer's cataract-knife), the edge upwards, in the sclerotic, about half a line from the corneal limbus, and near its upper and outer portion so that the anterior chamber will be opened across its extreme upper margin. Some operators enter at the junction of the cornea, and the sclerotic at a little lower point. The knife, being entered at the temporal side, is pushed downward and inward until it has entered the anterior chamber to the extent of two or three lines, when the handle is depressed and the point is carried horizontally forward towards the nasal margin of the cornea, so as to emerge in the sclerotic or limbus corneæ, exactly opposite its place of entrance; the edge of the blade is then turned sharply forwards, the knife pushed horizontally onward, and the section completed by drawing it backward from heel to point. The next step, the eye being steadied by an assistant, is to make an iridectomy by seizing the iris which presents itself at the wound, and snipping it off. The capsule is then lacerated, and, by gentle pressure upon the eye, the cataract is forced through the opening. If, as sometimes happens, the lens is not readily evacuated, it should be drawn from the eye by a small spoon-like tractor or curette.

SPOON EXTRACTION, OR THE TRACTION OPERATION.

The opening in this operation is made with the lance-shaped iridectomy-knife at the upper border of the cornea at its junction with the sclerotic, and enlarged laterally, when thought necessary, with the scissors. An iridectomy is then made, the capsule lacerated, and a scoop or miniature spoon is cautiously introduced, carried between the lens and posterior capsule, and the cataract slowly drawn from the eye.

There are many modifications of the flap and traction operations; but most of them are practised only by the inventors, and are not likely to be adopted to any extent by operators generally. Some of the modifications, such, for instance, as making an iridectomy some weeks previous to extraction will be useful in exceptional cases. Another modification, a combination of the flap and scoop operation, is for the purpose of

EXTRACTION OF THE LENS WITH CAPSULE.

A flap opening is made in the sclerotic or at the corneo-scleral junction, followed by an iridectomy; a scoop is then introduced behind the lens and capsule, and both are extracted together. Sometimes the lens in its capsule can be gently forced out by pressure alone. This form of extraction would seem to be indicated in cataract complicated by iritis or irido-choroiditis, as the lens being removed entire, no cortical portion remains, as in ordinary extraction, to excite inflammation.

RECLINATION OR DEPRESSION

For senile cataract has justly fallen into disrepute, and is seldom practised. It might sometimes be called for in very aged persons, unwilling to undergo the much severer operation of extraction. The eye is entered through the sclerotica, about two lines from the cornea at the temporal side, just below the horizontal meridian. The needle at present in use is delicate, flattened, and spear-shaped towards its point, and double-edged. It is carried forward until its flat surface is directly behind the pupil, and against the anterior capsule. The lens is then pressed gently backward and downward out of the field of vision. It is pressed in this particular direction in order that, if possible, it may lie isolated in the vitreous humor, free from contact with the ciliary bodies and the choroid, upon which it would otherwise act as a foreign body, and cause irritation. In fact, the great danger from the operation always is, that, sooner or later, the lens will come in contact with the choroidea and cause a choroiditis. Its effects are brilliant at first, but not permanent. Now and then there is an exceptionally successful result. I saw, during the semester of 1863, in Vienna, a man who had reclination performed for cataract in the year 1839, and now, for the first time, was troubled by indistinct vision from a shred of opaque capsule.

AFTER TREATMENT IN EXTRACTION.

After the operation both eyes should be gently closed and a simple bandage applied, as described in chapter second under Bandaging. The bandage and charpie should be removed twice a day, the discharge gently washed away with tepid water, and a soft moist sponge drawn across the edges of the tarsi, which frequently adhere to each other. Attentions of this kind render the patient more comfortable, quiet, and less nervous, and so facilitate healing and a fortunate result. The patient should keep his bed about forty-eight hours, and then if all goes well he may exchange it for the sofa. The bandage may be continued for ten or twelve days, and then be replaced by a broad shade, and the sooner after this the patient can get into the open air the better. The diet for the first day or day and a half may consist of farinaceous articles and beef-tea, but after this, should be generous, and nearly that to which he is accustomed. I always administer aconite after the operation for thirty-six hours or more. In case of constipation, later, bry. and nux are better than the "mild purgative" so often recommended by surgeons. If the eye is quite hot and painful during the first few hours after the extraction, cold compresses may be used. For the first forty-eight hours when the pain is severe, and the eyelids swollen with muco-purulent discharge, we may expect more or less *suppuration of the cornea.* A compress bandage is to be applied, and the case treated as described under Suppurative Corneitis and Ophthalmitis. This dangerous complication avoided, we may have an *acute iritis.* Atropine should be instilled into the eye at once, of the strength of four grains to the ounce of water, not only for the purpose of securing immobility to the iris, but to prevent if possible closure of the pupil. The advent of acute iritis may be known by pain, photophobia, lachrymation, chemosis, discoloration of the iris, turbid aqueous humor, and contracted pupil. The treatment of iritis has been already given. Simple iritis, of a serous character, may come on later from irritation of the iris, and is much less dangerous than the more rare *acute suppurative* or *traumatic* iritis, above mentioned. *Prolapse of the iris* is liable to occur soon after extraction, in which case atropine and the compress bandage are to be immediately applied. *Corneal fistula* from imperfect union of the lips of the wound will require the same treatment. If after two or three weeks no perfect union occurs, the edges of the orifice may be touched cautiously with a solution of arg. nit., which will probably effect the object through the local inflammation set up by it. If this fail, an iridectomy to relieve intraocular pressure should be tried. *Cystoid cicatrix*, the name given by Von Graefe to a healing of the wound in the sclera or limbus corneæ through the intervention of cicatricial tissue, which finally becomes thin and bulging, is noticed oftenest as a sequel of iridectomy for glaucoma. It may occur also in glaucomatous eyes after extraction. We cannot change the nature of the cicatrix, but we may perhaps prevent an increase of bulging, sometimes, by operating to remove intraocular pressure.

CAPSULAR OPACITIES AFTER EXTRACTION.

After fully dilating the pupil with atropine, the wrinkled, semi-opaque capsule which sometimes remains in the pupillary area, is to be torn open with a fine needle which is passed into the eye through the cornea. It may be necessary to use two needles, one in each hand, entered at opposite sides of the cornea; their points, meeting in the capsule can be moved in opposite directions, which renders the division of it easier and more certain. In some instances it cannot be torn by needles, and then it may be advisable to attempt the withdrawal of the tough capsule by means of the delicate canular forceps. It is a very hazardous proceeding, and I have often known it to fail. None of these operations should be undertaken until all irritability of the iris has passed away, and after the operation atropine should be instilled, bell. and acon. administered, and the patient kept for twenty-four hours in a subdued light.

SECONDARY CATARACT

Is an opacity of the lens occurring in the course of glaucoma and other deep-seated diseases of the eye. As a rule, no operation for the removal of the cataract is indicated, as the risk is very great, without a prospect of corresponding benefit, if all goes well. The operation of mine, following an iridectomy for glaucoma, published in the "New England Medical Gazette" for June, 1869, was unusually successful, more so perhaps than could have reasonably been hoped for. In that case, however, there were pretty certain indications that the fundus of the eye had been restored to a tolerably healthy condition. The patient could see a lighted candle in a darkened room at a distance of fifteen feet. There was evidence that the glaucoma had ceased to progress, and there was a chance, that whatever improvement of sight might be gained by the removal of the opaque lens, might be permanently retained.

SOFT CATARACT

Occurs in younger subjects, those under thirty-five or forty years of age. Its color and general appearance has already been noticed. One of the commonest forms of this lenticular opacity is the *infantile* or *congenital cataract.* It is either congenital, or develops during infancy. There are two varieties: the *lamellar*, called by German writers *schichtstaar*, is a central opacity surrounded by a more or less transparent zone of lens substance, so that when the pupil is fully dilated the sight is usually improved to a remarkable degree. It seems to be connected in some manner with infantile convulsions. The progress of the opacity is slow, sometimes almost imperceptibly so. Children with this form of cataract are often thought to be near-sighted. This idea may be corrected at once by the test mentioned under Amblyopia, and the cataract diagnosed by lateral illumination or the ophthalmoscope. The other variety of opacity, *the cortical cataract,* is much more rapid in its course. This opacity is seen in the form of opaque striæ running from the circumference to the centre, the interstices at first being of transparent lens, which after a time becomes mottled, hazy, and opaque.

When mature, the cataract is bluish-white, more dense at the centre, the striæ often presenting a pearly aspect. In infantile cataract an early operation is indicated in order to prevent, as far as possible, the amblyopia retinæ, which develops rapidly in young eyes, when the visual rays of light are excluded by opacities in the transparent media.

OPERATIONS FOR SOFT CATARACT.

The operations for soft cataract are those of *discission*, *linear extraction*, and *suction*. *Discission*, or *solution*, consists in entering the eye through the cornea with a fine needle, rupturing the capsule of the lens centrally, and lacerating more or less the lens substance, permitting its absorption by the aqueous humor, which obtains access to it through the opened capsule. Before the operation the pupil should be dilated with atropine, and subsequent to it, should be kept as widely dilated as possible, to avoid contact with lens matter, which might occasion otherwise irritation, possibly iritis. Several operations of puncturing or lacerating with the needle will be required before the whole of the substance of the opaque lens will be absorbed. The interval between each operation will probably be three months or more, according to the progress of absorption; whenever progress ceases the operation is to be repeated. Too much lens matter should not be broken up at once, lest too much swelling of the lens substance ensue, causing great irritation. If this should happen, the lens may be immediately removed from the eye by linear extraction. After the operation the patient should remain quiet for a day or two in a partially darkened room.

Iridodesis, or *iridectomy*, for an artificial pupil, is sometimes done for lamellar cataract, when it appears to be stationary or non-progressive. This affords very good vision if the circumference of the lens is clear and the opacity pretty sharply defined. It is, perhaps, the freest from danger of all operations, but if the cataract prove to be progressive and the opacity extends, the eccentric pupil is no longer serviceable, and the eye is perhaps not in quite so favorable condition for the most successful results from discission or linear extraction.

LINEAR EXTRACTION

Should be performed a few days subsequent to a needle operation, in which the laceration of the capsule and division of the substance of the lens, is more thorough and extended than in the one advised for discission and removal of the cataract by absorption. When the lens matter has become softened and swollen by admixture with the aqueous humor, the pupil being widely dilated by atropine, the cornea is opened at its temporal margin with a broad needle in an oblique direction. A curette is then introduced, the eye being fixed in the most convenient position with the forceps, and by gentle pressure upon the lips of the wound the semi-fluid lens will flow gently down the groove of the curette, and be brought out at the small corneal aperture. Afterwards the simple bandage should be applied, and the patient kept in bed for twenty-four or forty-eight hours, the pupil being dilated by atropine, applied daily, until all signs of iritis have disappeared.

THE SUCTION OPERATION,

Like the linear, is probably more easily accomplished a few days after breaking up the lens with the needle, although either operation may follow immediately, if necessary. The operation is like the last described, only in place of the ordinary curette, is substituted a tubular one, attached to a second tube, of glass, and this to a metal syringe, from which the suction power is obtained. The syringe is constructed so as to be worked by the right hand, which also guides the curette, while the left keeps the eye in position by the forceps.

Diabetic cataract, appearing in the course of a diabetes, is generally soft, but harder in elderly persons. It is to be removed by linear extraction, if the health of the patient is not too much impaired.

Fluid cataract is of rare occurrence. Generally there is a nucleus more or less firm. Suction or linear extraction, is the suitable operation for it. In appearance, it is milky-white, homogeneous, and without opalescent stripes.

TREATMENT OF CATARACT BY PARACENTESIS.

Sperino's method consists in repeatedly tapping the anterior chamber through the cornea, evacuating the aqueous several times at one sitting, and repeating the operation at frequent intervals an indefinite number of times; he operates twenty, fifty, a hundred times or more, on the same eye before the lens regains its transparency, and frequently this result is not attained in the end. The idea is, to permit the opaque fibres of the lens to regain their transparency through the relief to the intraocular circulation afforded by the paracentesis.

MEDICAL TREATMENT OF CATARACT.

It does not seem improbable to me that in the course of time, we may find some reliable remedy, the administration of which before the lens-fibre has become degenerated, may restore its transparency. Cataract is known to be a result of ergotism. It has also been produced in frogs by administering sugar in large quantities, or by injecting it under the skin. Chloride of sodium and alcohol have produced similar results. In our school, cures, or beneficial results, are reported to have followed the use of cannab., con., phosph., silex, sulph., and a few other of our remedies.

CAPSULAR CATARACT.

Opacity of the substance of the capsule probably never occurs by itself. There is always a previous opacity of the lens.

Anterior capsular cataract, or *false cataract*, is usually situated centrally, and is caused originally by an inflammation of the iris or cornea. In young children the anterior chamber is very shallow, and in the new-born it scarcely exists at all, the cornea and lens being nearly in contact, so that an ophthalmia would be likely to extend to the capsule, or, if purulent leave some deposit upon its anterior surface. When this opacity is prominent, and extends somewhat into the pupil, it has been called *pyramidal cataract*. An artificial pupil is usually indicated in this form of opacity. In *capsulo-lenticular cataract*, both capsule and lens are extracted either separately or together.

DISLOCATION OF THE LENS

May be spontaneous, the result of a blow on the eye or head, or it may be congenital and hereditary. It is either *partial* or *complete*. The lens may be thrown backwards into the vitreous humor, forward through the pupil into the anterior chamber, or by a rupture of the sclerotic it may be forced beneath the conjunctiva. In the latter case, and also when dislocated into the anterior chamber, it should be extracted. If lying in the vitreous it may be permitted to remain, if its presence occasions no great irritation, if otherwise, it should be extracted by the traction operation.

DIAGNOSIS.

There is generally pain, photophobia, lachrymation, tremulousness of the iris, and the signs of absence of the lens behind the pupil, mentioned under Aphakia. Lying in the anterior chamber the lens may be plainly seen and recognized. Not long since, however, a case was sent me which had been called an opacity of the cornea. It was in an eye otherwise diseased, and the dislocation was occasioned by a blow on the head. Under the conjunctiva, the displaced lens may be seen as a small semi-transparent swelling. In partial dislocations there will be monocular diplopia or polyopia. *Lateral illumination* will enable us to determine the amount of displacement. *Direct examination* with the ophthalmoscope is still better. We may then see the free edge of the lens as a dark crescentic line across the red pupil. Partial displacement often causes great irritation, and may lead to glaucomatous inflammation. In such cases the lens is to be extracted. Sometimes the great irritation experienced at first may be lessened by the instillation of atropine, by warm soothing fomentations of bell., cham., opium, and the internal administrations of acon., bell., cham., or, when the pain is deep seated, of spigel., macrot., or sanguin. In congenital or other cases, where the dislocation appears fixed, an operation for artificial pupil is indicated.

TRAUMATIC CATARACT.

The opacity in the lens generally commences within twenty-four hours after the injury to the capsule. It is at first confined to the locality of the wound, but soon involves the entire lens, spreading more rapidly, the younger the subject. There may be considerable pain and irritation resulting from the wound in the cornea or laceration of the iris, or simply from the pressure of the swollen lens upon the iris. Traumatic cataract may occur from a blow, which, without the rupture of the external tunics of the eye, may nevertheless rend the capsule of the lens. The pupil should be kept dilated, and the medical treatment be similar to that mentioned in dislocation of the lens. After the irritation has subsided, if the absorption of the lens is found to be going on, there should be no surgical interference; but if the pain continues, tension of the globe is increased, the pinkish zone around the border is marked, and traumatic glaucoma is feared, the lens should be extracted.

APHAKIA,

Or absence of the crystalline lens, occurs after extraction, from complete dislocation, and after absorption of the lens. It may be recognized when the history of the case is not known, by the blackness of the pupil, diminished size of the anterior chamber, and tremulousness of the iris in case the latter has lost the support of the capsule also. The refraction of the eye is, of course, much changed. An emmetropic eye becomes hypermetropic, a hypermetropic eye more hypermetropic, a myopic eye less myopic, and the power of accommodation is gone. The spectacles suited to this condition of the eye are spoken of in the next chapter.

CHAPTER XIII.

SPECTACLES—ARTIFICIAL EYES.

SPECTACLES.

THE ordinary glasses for spectacles, in optical defects, are convex or concave *spherical*, except in astigmatism, when they are *cylindrical*, or a combination of both spherical and cylindrical. The nature and use of these glasses have already been sufficiently explained.

CATARACT GLASSES

Are thick convex lenses of great refractive power. After extraction of the crystalline lens the accommodative power of the eye is lost, and therefore two pairs of spectacles will be necessary, one for reading of about 2½-inch focus, and the other 4½-inch focus for distance. These numbers will vary somewhat according to the refractive state of the eye before operating, whether emmetropic, myopic, or hypermetropic. It is advisable also that the glasses should be small and encircled by a black ring of ebony or shell a quarter of an inch in width. Large glasses admit too much light into the eye, and cause a dazzling sensation. Sometimes a combination of cylindrical with the spherical glasses are requisite in order to afford sufficient acuteness of vision for the patient to read with comfort.

Cataract glasses should not be worn for some weeks after the operation; while much irritation remains it is better not to attempt the use of the eyes for near objects.

PANTOSCOPIC GLASSES,

Verres à double foyer, are sometimes called Franklin glasses from the fact that he wore such. The upper and lower half of each glass have different foci. If a myope becomes presbyopic the upper half of his glasses would be concave for distance, and the lower half convex to neutralize his presbyopia in reading.

PRISMATIC AND DECENTRED GLASSES.

Prismatic glasses are useful in aiding or exercising certain muscles of the eye, as explained under the article on Strabismus. Decentred lenses are so constructed that the wearer looks through an eccentric part instead of the centre. A convex lens, for instance, is so arranged that its centre lies a little to the inner side of the visual axis, in consequence of which a slight prismatic effect is produced.

EYE PROTECTORS.

Eye protectors made of curved blue glass are the best. Goggles with wire, silk, or glass sides keep the eye, as a general rule, too close and warm. For photophobia, simple blue spectacles of plain glass are generally sufficient, and may be darker or lighter in shade, according to the amount of protection required. Brown or smoke-colored glasses may be used, if preferred. The latter cut off all the rays of light, and consequently render vision somewhat less distinct, while blue glasses, excluding the orange rays only, interfere less with the clear definition of objects. Green glasses protect the eye from the red rays alone; but it is the orange rays which are most intolerable to a sensitive retina.

Strong plate glass spectacles are worn by those finding it necessary to protect the eyes against chips and particles of stone or steel. It is proposed to make them of curved mica. Such spectacles would be cheap, durable, not likely to break, and very light.

STENOPAIC SPECTACLES,

Composed of metallic plates with small central apertures, are useful in opacities or cloudiness of the cornea. They exclude the peripheral, and permit only the central rays of light to enter the eye.

Acuteness of vision for near objects is increased, but they are not serviceable for more distant views, as they limit the field of vision too much.

ARTIFICIAL EYES.

After enucleation or excision of the eyeball, or after excision of a staphyloma of the cornea, or in case of a shrunken globe from any operative interference or disease, the deformity may be almost completely removed by wearing a suitable artificial eye. It should not be worn for a month or six weeks after the removal of the eyeball, lest irritation and inflammation of the conjunctiva ensue. To insert it, the upper lid is to be raised, the upper border of the artificial eye introduced beneath it, and the lid allowed to fall; then the lower lid is to be depressed and gently pulled forward when the artificial eye will slip into place. To remove it, depress the lower lid, and with a hook or bodkin force its lower edge forward, and it will fall out. It should be caught on something soft or yielding so as not to break or scratch it. It should be removed and cleansed every night, and, if worn every day, after six months should be exchanged for a new one, as at the end of this time it becomes roughened and may occasion irritation and inflammation.

CHAPTER XIV.

THE MUSCLES OF THE EYE.

PARALYSIS.

THE nerves supplying the muscles of the eye are the third, fourth, and sixth. The third supplies the internal, superior and inferior recti, the inferior oblique, the levator palpebræ superioris, the constrictor pupillæ, and the ciliary muscle.

The fourth nerve supplies the superior oblique, and the sixth the external rectus.

The rectus externus moves the eye outward.
" " internus moves the eye inward.
" " superior moves the eye upward and inward, and rolls (inclines the vertical meridian) the eye inward.
" " inferior moves the eye downward and inward, and rolls it outward.
" superior oblique moves the eye downward and outward, and rolls it inward.
" inferior oblique moves the eye upward and outward, and rolls it outward.

The third and sixth nerves are more often affected, the fourth very rarely. For convenience in describing the diagnostic symptoms, we will consider the paralytic affection as occurring in the left eye.

PARALYSIS OF THE EXTERNAL RECTUS.

On moving an object before the eye from right to left (a lighted candle is convenient), a convergent squint is noticed. The movement of the eye to the left is sluggish. There is diplopia as the object is moved into the left half of the field of vision, the images being homonymous (not crossed, the right belonging to the right eye, the left to the left eye), parallel, of the same height, the distance between them increasing as the object is moved further to the left. The position of the head is also characteristic, the patient carrying it turned somewhat to the left, in order to avoid the confusion of sight arising from the double images. A prismatic glass may be worn to correct the diplopia.

A prism bends the rays of light towards its base. Applying it to the left eye, base towards the temple, rays of light are bent outward, and the image is projected inward towards that of the other eye. The prismatic glass should be just strong enough to fuse the two images. If we wish to exercise the paralyzed rectus so as gradually to strengthen it, we may prescribe a weaker prismatic glass which does not quite fuse, but approximates very nearly the two images. The effort of the eye to fuse the images will call the rectus externus into action to a limited extent, and as it grows stronger we may weaken the strength of the prism.

PARALYSIS OF THE INTERNAL RECTUS

Is rarely met with as an isolated affection. The third nerve, supplying also the superior and inferior recti, the inferior oblique and others, several muscles are simultaneously affected. The symptoms would, however, be the reverse of those just noticed, and prismatic glasses would be worn with the base inward. The patient would also incline his head slightly towards the right. In

PARALYSIS OF THE SUPERIOR RECTUS,

The eye will not turn upwards readily. There is also a slight divergent squint. The inferior oblique drawing the eye outward, crossed double images will occur in the upper half of the visual field. The images are not parallel, diverge upwards, and differ in height.

PARALYSIS OF THE INFERIOR RECTUS

Would occasion symptoms just the reverse of the above. In

PARALYSIS OF THE SUPERIOR OBLIQUE

The deviation of the visual axis is but very slight. There is a want of mobility noticed in the attempt to turn the eye downwards and inwards. Homonymous, or corresponding double images are seen in the lower half of the field of vision. The left image (that of the affected eye) appears lower than the other. The images will be oblique, converging towards the top. The patient will be annoyed in descending stairs, which appear double, and irregular in outline. He will be apt to turn his head downward and to the right, so as to bring objects into the upper and left portion of the field of vision, avoiding the diplopia. Prisms are worn base downward and outward.

PARALYSIS OF THE THIRD NERVE

May be complete, affecting all the muscles supplied by it, or it may be partial, affecting only one or more of the muscles. In complete paralysis, say, of the left eye, there is first ptosis. On raising the upper lid we find the eye restricted in its movements in the upward, downward, and inward directions. The rectus externus, being supplied by the sixth nerve, is unaffected, and the eye can consequently move outward. It can also move to a certain extent downward and outward, through the superior oblique, which is supplied by the fourth nerve.

PROGNOSIS AND TREATMENT.

Whether a cure of paralysis of the muscles of the eye can be prognosed, depends chiefly upon the cause of the affection. If syphilitic, a not uncommon cause, the prognosis is generally favorable. If of rheumatic origin, the prognosis is highly favorable. When due to intracranial causes, the prognosis is, of course, often unfavorable. The more acute the case, generally speaking, the better are the chances for a cure. In syphilitic cases, I believe iodide of potash, after merc., to be the best remedy. In rheumatic cases, where the seat of the disease is the sheath of the nerve, my experience has been excellent with bry. Gelsem., merc., macrot., nux, ignat., and other remedies, have appeared more or less beneficial. The chances of cure are much increased if the paralysis is partial and only one nerve affected, the general nervous system being in good condition. In case of paralysis of the sixth nerve (external rectus), the condition of the abdominal viscera should receive more than ordinary attention, as this nerve seems to be particularly influenced by reflex action from the sympathetic. When other means fail, paralysis of the ocular muscles from peripheral or extracranial causes may frequently be cured by electricity. Faradization does not appear to be as efficacious as the primary galvanic current. Benedict * had unusual facilities for testing the value of electricity at the clinics of Prof. Arlt, in Vienna. Of twenty-seven cases, all but five were benefited, and seventeen of them cured. Contrary to the generally received opinion, which attributes the benefit to the direct excitation of the paralyzed nerve, he found "that the cure was dependent, generally speaking, upon reflex irritation through the fifth pair of nerves." He found further that "in most cases a curative action was only produced when the excitation was relatively weak." He used from three to fifteen of Daniell's elements. The excitation should only continue about *half a minute* at each sitting, the improvement occurring in most cases *instantaneously*. In operating, the copper pole is generally placed on the forehead, while the zinc pole is, in affection of the external rectus, placed over the cheek-bone, in ptosis over the affected lid, in paralysis of the internal rectus or the inferior oblique, over the side of the nose at the inner angle of the eye, in case of the inferior rectus, over the lower margin of the orbit, and in paralysis of the superior oblique, on the nose at the internal angle of the eye. In mydriasis, the zinc pole being on the cheek-bone,

* The interesting article on this subject from which my information is obtained, is in the "Ophthalmic Review," No. 6, page 143. It is a translation from the "Archiv. für Ophthalmologie."

the copper pole should be applied over the closed eyelid.

The prognosis, under any treatment, of cases arising from intracranial lesions is unfavorable. Pain in the head, dizziness, loss of intellectual power, unsteady movements, and great difficulty in fusing the double images by prisms, all indicate a cerebral cause. Among the cerebral lesions may be mentioned tubercular deposits, hydrocephalus, effusions of blood, aneurisms, softening of the brain and tumors. Ostitis, periostitis, exostosis, and tumors situated at the base of the brain, sometimes occasion the paralysis. Similar orbital affections may also cause it.

In children, oftener than in adults, a local paralysis may be the result of some nervous irritation in a distant part. Dentition is often the exciting cause, and in such instances the prognosis is nearly always favorable.

In adults the annoyance of the constant double vision is relieved by bandaging one eye, or by the use of spectacles, one glass of which may be dark or frosted.

SURGICAL TREATMENT.

When other remedial measures fail, or only partially complete the cure, the abnormal direction of the eye and the resulting diplopia may sometimes be remedied by an operation to restore the equilibrium of the muscles. The description of operations on the muscles of the eyeball is given under the article Strabismus.

PARALYSIS OF THE CILIARY MUSCLE

Is not of common occurrence. It has been noticed chiefly during convalescence from severe fevers and debilitating diseases like diphtheria. It may be produced temporarily by dropping a small quantity of a solution of sulphate of atropine, four or six grains to the ounce of water, into the eye. The patient sees well at a distance, but is not able to read fine print. Near objects appear indistinct. Suitable convex glasses will restore near vision.

Perfect rest of the eyes and frequent bathing in cold water should be enjoined. The diet in these cases ought to be generous and nutritious, and hygienic conditions should be made as favorable as possible. Remedies adapted to the impoverished condition of the patient's system, like china, ferrum, or hydras. will be indicated. Recovery is generally satisfactory.

SPASM OF THE CILIARY MUSCLE

Is sometimes met with in hypermetropia. It occasions myopic refraction of the eye, so that the patient sees better in the distance through concave glasses. By paralyzing the ciliary muscle, however, we find that the eye is really hypermetropic; the spasm appears to be the result of overworking the ciliary muscle in accommodating (see article Asthenopia and Hypermetropia). The affection may also be diagnosed by the aid of the ophthalmoscope, which shows a hypermetropic refraction notwithstanding the existing myopia for distance. The simple device of the card with the pinhole, mentioned under Amblyopia, may also be of use in diagnosis.

TREATMENT.

The eye should be allowed complete rest, and it may be necessary to paralyze the ciliary muscle by the daily instillation of atropine solution for some weeks, so as to insure complete rest to the ciliary muscle also. Internally, the general health of the patient being good, I would use nux v. and gels., from having used these remedies with good results in spasmodic affection of the orbicularis. The internal use of small doses of physostigma might also prove serviceable. The spasmodic affection being cured, the case should be treated as one of accommodative asthenopia.

Nystagmus, or involuntary oscillation of the eyeball, is owing to spasmodic twitching of the muscles which control the globe. It is most frequently seen in congenital cataract in children, but may be brought on by any affection of the eye which causes indistinctness of vision. Its cure can only be effected by restoring acuteness of vision to the diseased eye.

STRABISMUS (CONCOMITANT STRABISMUS).

When the eye is turned inward it is termed *convergent strabismus*, if outward *divergent strabismus*. If confined to one eye it is called *monocular*, if the squint alternates between the two eyes, it is *binocular* or *alternating strabismus*. In the latter case, the acuteness of vision in the two eyes being about the same, the patient fixes, sometimes one eye, sometimes the other, on the object, the squinting eye being the one not in use for the time being. In monocular strabismus the sight of the squinting eye is almost invariably impaired, and no attempt is made by the patient to use it.

In treatment it is practical to divide strabismus also into the *periodic* and the *confirmed*, although the pathology of the two is usually identical, and the first is but the precursor of the second. Occasionally, however, we meet with a periodic squint, especially in children, where the affection may be traced to some nervous irritation in a distant part, or to the cerebral irritation from dentition. No doubt that a squint of this kind arises often from partial paralysis of one or more of the ocular muscles, and is therefore not properly spoken of under the head of Concomitant Strabismus. In the latter there is a tension or an increased energy or shortening of a muscle, but the eyeball can be moved outward or inward at will, which is not the case in paralytic strabismus.

The commonest cause of concomitant strabismus is hypermetropia. It is caused also by myopia, and by amblypopia, corneal opacities, or any circumstance which renders vision of one eye defective.

CONVERGENT STRABISMUS

Is usually due to hypermetropia. Donders believes this to be the cause in seventy-seven per cent, and Wecker in eighty per cent. It will be remembered that in the hypermetropic eye the antero-posterior diameter is too short, and that parallel rays of light reach the retina before being focussed, and vision is therefore indistinct: that the refractive power of such eyes requires to be aided by convex glasses in order to prevent over-exertion in accommodating or *accommodative asthenopia*. In regarding near objects still greater exertions to accommodate are necessary, and consentaneous with accommodation comes the convergence of the visual axis in order to fix both eyes on the same near point. Convergence however in such eyes is greater, than under similar circumstances, it would be in normally refractive (emmetropic) eyes. A habit of turning the eyes inward is formed, which results first in a periodic, then in a permanent, squint. Such squint often makes its appearance in children at the age of four, five, or six years, when they are learning to read, and is often attributed to any cause but the right one. Sometimes its appearance is noticed a few years later, when the first earnest study is begun. If one eye happen to be more hypermetropic than the other, the tendency to squint is still stronger, for this eye may then turn inward without the annoyance which would otherwise be occasioned by the production of distinct double vision. The same would be true if in hypermetropia one eye happens to be amblyopic or defective in vision from opacity of any kind.

DIVERGENT STRABISMUS

Is very apt to be associated with myopia. Large staphyloma posticum, or posterior bulging of the globe, increases the tendency of the myopic eye to turn outward, as does also the frequent insufficiency of power in the internal recti met with in myopia. On account of the elongated shape of the eyeball it is almost impossible to turn both eyes inward so as to make their axes converge to the near point requisite for myopic vision. Therefore one eye is used and the other rolls outward. One eye being more myopic than the other increases the tendency to divergent strabismus. Great defects of sight in both eyes, vision being almost absent, are apt to produce slight divergent squint.

TO DETERMINE WHICH EYE IS AFFECTED.

Let the patient regard an object a few feet from him, then cover one eye with the hand, and note whether the uncovered eye has to make a lateral movement in order to fix itself on the object. We try each eye in this way, and the deviating eye is the affected one. This determines the *primary deviation.* The *secondary deviation* is the associated movement which the sound *covered* eye makes while the squinting eye is adjusting itself upon the object. The primary and secondary movements *are equal in extent.* This is an important fact in the differential diagnosis of ordinary or *concomitant* squint and *paralytic* squint. In the latter, the secondary deviation is the greater. Suppose the external rectus of the right eye paralyzed, and the eye turned inward. Hold an object before the eyes and covering the left, the right will move slowly outward, perhaps the distance of a line, in order to fix itself, while the associated movement of the covered eye, inward, will probably equal two or three lines; the reason of this is plain; the right externus is very weak, the left internus healthy; the impulse necessary to turn the right eye outward is much greater than is necessary for the associated movement of the left eye inward, — hence the greater movement of the left eye.

The amount of the deviation of a squinting eye, an important point to be considered in case of an operation, is found by marking with a pen the point on the lower lid directly beneath the centre of the pupil of the affected eye, while it is turned inward or outward, and then covering the sound eye permit the former to fix itself on some convenient object when a second mark beneath the centre of the pupil is again made. The distance between the two marks gives the extent of the strabismus. Several instruments are in vogue also for the measurement of squint, but the above method is simple, and generally sufficiently exact.

TREATMENT.

The treatment, of course, will depend very much upon the cause; also upon the history, duration, the state of vision, amount of deviation, periodicity or permanency, and whether monocular or binocular. All these points are first to be investigated.

When the squint is recent, and the result of nervous disturbance from ascarides, dentition, whooping-cough, gastric or other visceral affection, the removal of the primary disease by suitable medication may restore the eyes to their normal position. Many cures of this kind are recorded in our literature. Hirsch * publishes several cases dependent on helminthiasis, cured with spig., cina, sepia, and sulph. Cyclamen † cured a boy aged two and a half years, of strabismus of six months' standing, following convulsions. The same remedy also cured a child aged two and a half months, of squint following measles,‡ and also a coachman of Vienna. The particulars not given. Gallavardin § cured with hyos. a case of eight years' standing, in a girl of twelve, but failed in other cases. Afterwards, following the treatment of Tavignot, he cured two cases with phosph., it is said. The treatment with phosph. is probably better suited to cases of paralytic than concomitant squint. Gallavardin recommends alumin., bell., hyos.,‖ stram., and tabac.

Recent cases dependent on hypermetropia may often be cured by the use of convex glasses. The following is a case in point: Mr. B. called, on April 19, 1869, in consequence of a convergent strabismus

* "British Journal of Homœopathy," July, 1857, from the "Neue Zeitschrift für Homœopathische Klin."

† "American Homœopathic Review," Vol. II. p. 224.

‡ "Marcy and Hunt's Practice," Vol. II. p. 560.

§ "British Journal of Homœopathy," Appendix, 1860, p. 240.

‖ Jahr says: For this defect (disposition to squint) I give children, with the best result, hyos. or bell., in the first place, and if those do not help, alumin. — Ed. "Medical Investigator."

of the right eye, since two weeks. He had also severe asthenopia for a number of weeks, brought on from overuse of his eyes in book-keeping. His general health was perfect. I found a hypermetropia of about $\frac{1}{24}$, and prescribed convex glasses, at the same time cautioning him in regard to over-exertion of the eyes At the end of a week the squint, which at first was more than a line in extent, had nearly vanished, and in two weeks it was gone. The asthenopia was cured also.

The periodic, divergent squint, seen often in myopes, may frequently be cured by prescribing the proper concave glasses, so that they may see distant objects without effort.

Orthopædic exercise of the internus or externus muscle, when the deviation is not of great extent, is sometimes curative. The exercise is best accomplished by means of prisms, and presupposes tolerable sight in the affected eye. If this does not exist, bandaging the sound eye systematically for a short time every day, may, in a few weeks, restore sufficient vision for our purpose.

To correct a convergent squint the prism should be used with its base inward, thus inducing a corrective squint outward. The eye is turned outward through the involuntary effort to fuse the double images, care being taken that the prism be of just sufficient strength to nearly, but not quite, accomplish the fusion. In order to exercise the internal rectus the base of the prism should be directed outward. These orthopædic measures will generally be found more efficacious in paralytic than in concomitant squint. In the latter, however, they may be used to advantage, when necessary, in perfecting the result of an operation, and especially in aiding to fuse the double images, which sometimes are very annoying even after the most successful operations. Another method of treatment favorably mentioned for convergent strabismus dependent on hypermetropia, in children, is to paralyze the ciliary muscle with atropine, so as to prevent all attempts to accommodate up to the time when suitable glasses can be worn. Commenced early, during periodic squint, this treatment has proved successful.

SURGICAL TREATMENT OF STRABISMUS.

When the case is of long standing the operation of tenotomy is indicated, the object being to divide the shortened muscle at its insertion in the sclerotic, and permit it to reattach itself farther back.

The operation which I usually perform, and which I think most advisable, is that of Von Graefe. The eyelids having been separated by a speculum or an assistant, supposing it a case of convergent strabismus, the assistant turns the eye outward with a pair of forceps. The operator then seizes with delicate forceps a fold of the conjunctiva near the cornea, just below the middle line of the insertion of the internal rectus. Snipping it through with the scissors, he burrows underneath the conjunctiva somewhat, upward, downward, and inward, separating, to a limited extent, the subconjunctival tissue from the muscle. The strabismus hook is now inserted beneath the tendon at its lower edge to raise it from the globe and hold it, and the muscle is divided by a succession of delicate snips with the scissors *as near as possible* to its insertion in the sclerotic.

The operation is quite severe, but adults bear it readily without etherization. Children should be etherized. Very little after-treatment is required. If the eye is hot and painful, a cold compress may be applied over the closed lids, and a few doses of aconite administered. The divided muscle will reunite itself to the sclerotica within three or four days, and while this process is being accomplished it is well to bandage *the sound eye* so as to compel a central position for the other, and insure the attachment of the internus behind its former insertion. The daily or occasional exercise of the squinting eye, by bandaging the sound one, for some weeks before the operation, for the purpose of restoring acuteness of vision, when the eye is amblyopic from want of use for years, is commendable.

If the squint is of considerable extent it is better to operate on both eyes. For instance, if the strabismus is three lines in extent, by one operation on the affected eye we may reduce it to one line, then a slighter operation on the sound eye will bring the visual axes of both parallel. One operation will not usually remove more than from two to two and a half lines of deviation. The effect is increased by a free separation of subconjunctival tissue from the muscle when operating. The effect is decreased by avoiding this. The effect may also be increased *after* the operation by making the patient wear glasses, the right half of each glass being blackened with court-plaster (the left eye having been operated on), so that the affected eye is turned far outward during the process of healing; or, a thread may be inserted in the conjunctiva and the eye turned outward and held by attaching the thread to the cheek with adhesive plaster. The effect may be lessened when, after an operation, on testing the result we find that we have done too much, by inserting a conjunctival suture, bringing the edge of the wound, and with it the muscle, farther towards the cornea.

The operation of Liebreich* is similar to that of Graefe, except that he separates the subconjunc-

---

* See "Archives of Ophthalmology and Otology," No. 1, Vol. I. p. 26.

tival tissue back to the semi-lunar fold, and "divides the latter, likewise, as well as the caruncle, from the subadjacent parts," and "lengthens the vertical section of the capsule, above and below," and always closes the conjunctival wound with a suture. He claims that the effect of the operation in this way may be so increased that no more than one operation on one eye is ever necessary; that the sinking in of the caruncle, and the apparent bulging of the globe occasionally noticed, is avoided.

Usually the sinking in of the caruncle, and the accompanying undue prominence in the globe, formerly noticed after operations for strabismus, are to be avoided by limiting the separation of the subconjunctival fascia with the scissors, avoiding, also, all unnecessarily large excursions with the hook, and, above all, by being careful to divide the *tendon* of the muscle at its insertion, rather than the muscle itself farther back.

In rare instances, both in paralytic and concomitant squint, it becomes necessary to advance the insertion of a muscle so as to give it greater power. The operations mostly practised are those of Critchett, Graefe, and Liebreich, for the descriptions of which I am obliged to refer the reader to the larger works on Ophthalmology.

CHAPTER XV.

THE EYELIDS.

BLEPHARITIS, OR OPHTHALMIA TARSI,

Is a follicular inflammation of the edges of the lids, which are red and swollen. Excessive secretion from the follicles of the cilia produces a morning agglutination of the lids in the beginning, and later, in severe cases, the discharge becomes purulent, there are pustules and superficial ulceration, the cilia fall out, the tarsal border becomes thickened and rounded, the lids are crusted, the puncta lachrymalia no longer catch the tears, and the excoriation and irritation of the edge of the lids are kept up by their constant overflow. The cause of the affection in mild cases may be overuse of the eyes, especially in an unwholesome atmosphere, and such causes, generally, as tend to produce a hyperæmia of the conjunctiva. Severe cases occur mostly in ill-fed and ill-housed scrofulous subjects, and often as a sequence of ophthalmia scrofulosa, or of exanthematous fever.

TREATMENT.

In mild cases, rest of the eyes, avoidance of impure atmosphere, the application to the edge of the tarsi at night of simple cerate, or of an unguent of one grain of white precipitate to a drachm of simple cerate, and the administration of merc., internally, will suffice to cure. In severe cases, in bad subjects, we must rely chiefly on the constitutional means mentioned under Conjunctivitis Scrofulosa. The name of the unguents recommended for these cases is legion, but I find one better and simpler than the others, and generally as effective as can be expected for an inflammation which is to be regarded merely as a local manifestation of a constitutional disease. It is made of two grains of the red precipitate to a drachm of simple cerate; a small portion is rubbed between the cilia or along the edge of the tarsi at night, and in conjunction with this the red oxide of mercury in the second or third trituration, is administered internally. As an intercurrent remedy, an unguent of pot. iod. two grains, to the drachm of cerate, with kali hydriod., internally, I have also used with more or less benefit. Cleanliness must be rigidly insisted on, the crusts must be soaked off with tepid water, or milk and water, every morning, or no treatment will avail much. For excoriated lids from overflow of the tears or eczema, a lotion of ten grains of borax to the ounce of water, to which a few drops of glycerine may be added, or a solution of one grain of the acetate of lead to an ounce of water, with the addition of a few drops of glycerine, will be grateful to the exposed surface, and prove useful at least, as a palliative. In such cases slitting up the canaliculus, as directed in the next chapter, will often aid the tears in finding their proper channel. Other internal remedies are those recommended in Scrofulous Ophthalmia.

ACNE CILIARIS

Is a similar, but much milder, inflammation of the hair follicles at the edge of the lid. It appears mostly in youthful persons in conjunction with acne of the face, and is due to the same causes, and requires the same internal and dietetic treatment. The lids should be carefully cleansed every morning. I have found sepia and sulph. the most efficient remedies.

HERPES ZOSTER FRONTALIS. (SEU OPHTHALMICUS.)

A number of affections of the eye have been observed associated with herpes zoster frontalis. Among them are conjunctivitis, corneitis, ulceration of the cornea, iritis, paralysis of the third nerve, and the ophthalmic branch of the fifth. It has been noticed that unless the vesicles spread to the nose, the eye usually escapes all complication in the disease; and that the affection of the eye is generally most severe when the vesicles extend downward to the tip of the nose. The treatment of the eye will be mostly palliative, and such as has been given in this work in its proper place. The cure will depend upon the removal of the herpes zoster by the means and remedies laid down in the works of our school on General Practice. The prognosis in such cases is good, except in old and feeble subjects.

MALPOSITION OF THE LIDS.

ECTROPIUM, EVERSION OF THE EYELIDS,

May be caused by the various ophthalmiæ, and by cicatrices from injuries. Arlt, of Vienna, used to advise us in these cases to bandage the eye, the indication being to shorten the lids and to protect the exposed mucous surface from the air. The pressure is to be made by means of charpie and the bandage, not upon the eyeball, but at the angles of the lid, chiefly at the inner angle, so as to increase the tension of the orbicularis. After three or four days the improvement will be decided, provided the bandage has been readjusted whenever displaced.

ENTROPIUM, INVERSION OF THE LID,

Is due generally to old purulent or granular ophthalmia, in which, both from the disease, and the improper use of caustics, structural changes of the conjunctiva have resulted. It is sometimes due, in the lower lid, to a spasmodic affection. *Trichiasis*, the turning inward of the eyelashes, and the consequent irritation of the surface of the cornea, is a usual feature of this affection. *Distichiasis*, a double row of cilia, more or less regularly placed, results also from old ophthalmiæ. The cilia may be extracted in these cases with the cilia forceps. The simple excision of a fold of the skin beneath the lower lid will sometimes remove the entropium. In the treatment of ectropium and entropium, the palliative measures mentioned for ophthalmia tarsi and the medical and hygienic treatment recommended for scrofulous ophthalmia will always be indicated. In severe cases surgical means will be required also. For the multitude of operations suited to the various phases of these affections, I am reluctantly obliged to refer the reader to the more comprehensive surgical works. Syphilitic and cancerous ulcerations of the lid, the latter being usually of the rodent or epithelial variety, require the same medical treatment as if situated elsewhere. I have no new experiences to offer. A case of rodent cancer of the lid, now under my treatment for about six weeks, and of several years' standing, is improving under arsen., internally, and Simpson's paste, externally.

TUMORS OF THE EYELIDS.

CHALAZION, OR MEIBOMIAN CYST,

Is a morbid enlargement of a meibomian gland, generally isolated and in the upper lid, but sometimes found in the lower lid, and sometimes a number are noticed in one lid at the same time. They are recognized at first as small hard prominences which, as they grow larger, gradually become softer. The contents are gelatinous, or semi-fluid, occasionally nearly fluid. Such tumors are usually an indication of impaired health. Mothers are frequently subject to them after confinement and nursing.

TREATMENT.

These tumors, in rare instances, disappear without treatment. I have known several instances of the kind. Occasionally I have succeeded in curing them promptly by administering merc., internally, and permitting the application night and morning, to the external face of the tumor, of an unguent of four or six grains of red precipitate to the ounce of cerate. They may sometimes be cured by restoring the general health of the patient by medical and hygienic means, but oftener than otherwise, it will be necessary to reverse the lid, make a small incision over the inner surface of the tumor and squeeze out the contents, or remove them with a small spoon or curette. The operation may be performed without etherization, and, by applying the eyelid tourniquet, may be rendered almost bloodless. The tumor is liable to recur, and constitutional remedies should be used to prevent this.

OTHER TUMORS OF THE LIDS

Are the *sebaceous*, or *dermoid*, which appear at the upper and outer margin of the orbit, but sometimes at the lower and inner, and when annoying are to be dissected out. Probably no medical means will suffice for their removal. Milium or molluscum, small white tumors, are to be pricked or incised, and their contents squeezed out. *Nævi*, and *aneurisms by anastomosis*, are to be treated as in other parts of the body. *Warts* may be ligatured or snipped off with the scissors.

HORDEOLUM, OR STYE,

Is a small boil at or near the margin of the lid. It is rarely necessary to lance it. At the commencement if the fever and pain are considerable, cold compresses and acon. are indicated, otherwise puls., followed by staph., is usually the best treatment. If dependent on general debility of the patient the disease will be likely to recur unless the general health is restored. *Abscess of the lid* is generally the result of injury. The treatment will be precisely the same as for abscess in other parts of the body. In case lancing is necessary the incision should be made in a horizontal direction, so that the cicatrix remaining will be scarcely noticeable.

EPICANTHUS

Is a crescentic fold of skin overlapping the inner canthi of the eyes, giving the face in this region an Asiatic aspect. Operations are undertaken solely for cosmetic considerations, and although successful up to the point perhaps of rendering the nationality of the subject doubtful, cannot always be said to enhance the charms of such faces to the extent desired by near relatives. I remember a case of epicanthus at Sichel's Clinic, in Paris, in a girl six or seven years of age. Sichel advised pinching up the skin at the bridge of the nose with the fingers, "ten or twenty times a day for five minutes." The deformity is congenital, and decreases as the child grows older. The operation for it consists in excising vertical folds of skin in the spaces between the eyes and uniting the edges of the wound with sutures.

PARALYSIS OF THE ORBICULARIS, — LAGOPHTHALMOS,

Prevents complete closure of the lids. After a time the eye becomes irritable from constant exposure; lachrymation, conjunctivitis, corneitis, and other evils follow. If the cause of the disease is peripheral, from exposure to cold or dampness, bry., macrot., merc., colch., and similar remedies, will be indicated. The eye should always be shaded, or lightly covered. For the treatment when due to central or cerebral causes, see Treatment of Paralysis of Muscles of the Eye.

SPASM OF THE ORBICULARIS, OR BLEPHAROSPASM,

Is met most frequently in scrofulous ophthalmia. It is a spasmodic closure of the lids, associated with affections of the eyes where considerable photophobia is present. It is met with in purulent and granular ophthalmias, corneitis, iritis, hyperæsthesia of the retina, in supraorbital neuralgias, and in cases of foreign body in the eye. With the removal of the above affections, the nature and treatment of which are spoken of elsewhere, the spasm of the orbicularis ceases.

Sometimes the disposition to spasmodic closure of the lids becomes chronic, and long and patient treatment is necessary to effect a cure. I have a case now under treatment of a year and a half standing. It is caused by a hyperæmia and hyperæsthesia of the retina. The patient has been under treatment three months, is now much improved, and will, I think, eventually be cured. I began with the administration of nux v. rather than cactus, gelsem., macrot., and spigel., remedies which I often found useful in similar irritations of the nervous structure of the eye, chiefly on account of some general nervous debility, a slight frontal headache, and want of appetite. The nux v. was followed by gels. internally and externally (ten drops of the tincture to half a cup of water, for bathing the lids), and this has proved even more useful than the nux, *relieving the photophobia remarkably.* The patient is now so much better that I am certain that these two remedies will cure the case. Medium smoke-colored glasses were prescribed for out-of-door use. Occasionally, in severe neuralgia, when the spasm can be relieved by pressure over a branch of the fifth nerve, the branch has been divided by incision, and the disease cured. *Nictitation*, a slight convulsive twitching, or too frequent winking or blinking of the lids, is often noticed in very nervous or hysterical individuals. It often accompanies other nervous debility, is greatly increased by mental agitation, is sometimes under control through great effort, and at other times quite involuntary. It is often incurable, but may sometimes be removed by improving the condition of the nervous system of the patient. It is occasionally an indication of defective refraction of the eye, and is then cured by supplying the patient with the proper spectacles.

PTOSIS,

Or drooping of the upper lid, may be due to paralysis of the third nerve, or of the branch which supplies the levator muscle. In such instances the treatment should, in the main, be that laid down for paralysis of the ocular muscles. Gels., spig., zinc., plumb., and nux, will of course be thought of as acting specifically upon the levator palpebræ superioris.

The disease is sometimes congenital, and sometimes the result of injury. An operation may be performed for its relief, but is not advisable unless the ptosis is nearly or quite complete, and occasions great inconvenience. The best operation is that for the subcutaneous contraction of the upper lid. A transverse incision is made along the margin of the lid, about two and a half lines from its edge. The lips of the wound being drawn apart, the integument is dissected from the orbicularis until the latter is sufficiently exposed. A horizontal strip of the muscle three or four lines in width is then excised, and the wound closed by sutures, which pass through the skin and the cut edges of the orbicularis.

Cases of partial ptosis in feeble persons from tumefaction of the lid due to effusion beneath the skin are not unfrequent, and are to be relieved only by such general measures as the impaired health demands.

CHAPTER XVI.

THE LACHRYMAL APPARATUS.

EPIPHORA,

Or the excessive secretion of tears, is due to some mechanical irritation of the eye like that of a foreign body, an inverted eyelash, to a conjunctivitis or ophthalmia, and to deep-seated inflammations of the eye. It is frequently a reflex nervous symptom in mental emotion and in various disorders of the general nervous system. The treatment must, of course, be directed to the removal of the irritation. It is perhaps doubtful whether hypersecretion of tears, due to functional disorder of the lachrymal gland, and independent of affections of the eye, ever exists. Profuse lachrymation is not a symptom of any of the recognized diseases of this gland.

STILLICIDIUM LACHRYMARUM,

Or the ordinary "watery eye," is an entirely different affection, and may always be suspected when one eye alone is affected, and no immediate cause of irritation is present. It arises from an obstruction to the flow of tears through the lachrymal passage. Finding no exit, the tears collect along the margin of the lower lid, and finally drop slowly over its edge upon the cheek. The lid, after some time, becomes red and swollen from this constant moisture, and we have a monocular blepharitis or ophthalmia tarsi. When the lower puncta have become everted or obliterated so as no longer to catch the tears, the punctum and canaliculus are to be slit up, thus converting the outlet into an open channel.

SLITTING THE CANALICULUS

Is a very simple operation, but by no means as easy as simple. I generally dilate the orifice somewhat with a delicate probe, and then putting the lid slightly upon the stretch, slit the canal with a pair of fine sharp-pointed scissors. Many operators insert a fine grooved director, and using it for a guide, slit the canal with a cataract knife. Others use a probe-pointed knife, or probe-pointed scissors, and still others, the instrument of Giraud Teulon, combining the grooved director and a spring knife. No assistant is necessary unless the patient is unusually timid or very young. If the lower punctum happen to be obliterated, it may be necessary to pass a fine probe around into its canal by the way of the upper punctum in order to determine its exact position before attempting to lay it open. Many surgeons in France and Germany prefer opening the upper canaliculus as affording a more direct way to the sac. When the upper lid is drawn well back, the direction of the canaliculus is almost in a line with the direction of the sac, and the abrupt change of the probe from the horizontal to the vertical position, necessary when passing it from the lower canaliculus, is avoided. The upper canal is best slit with a delicate probe-pointed knife like Weber's.

In rare instances the canaliculus may be obstructed by a foreign body, such as an eyelash, or a minute chalky concretion, the removal of which effects a cure of the case.

ACUTE INFLAMMATION OF THE LACHRYMAL SAC

Comes on rapidly, and is often mistaken for erysipelas of the face. The region about the inner angle of the eye is exquisitely sensitive to touch, the lids are red and œdematous, and the inflammation and pain over the sac are intense until it bursts, when complete relief ensues. The cause of inflammations and suppurations of this kind is very likely a previous obstruction to the flow of tears. Retention of the lachrymal secretion in the sac gives rise to dilatation and hypertrophy, and favors the formation of abscess. Repeated suppuration leads to complete obstructions of the passage, to lachrymal fistula, and to disease of the lachrymal or superior maxillary bone. Nasal polypi sometimes obstruct the lachrymal passage. The treatment of these diseases of the lachrymal duct and sac will necessarily be mechanical as well as medical and topical.

TREATMENT OF ACUTE INFLAMMATION OF THE SAC.

Acon. and bell., in this affection, will be required internally, with cold, or perhaps ice-water, compresses externally. By these means the formation of abscess and bursting of the sac, or the necessity of lancing the sac, are frequently averted. Another means of averting perforation is to slit the upper canaliculus, and passing down a narrow knife incise the neck of the sac, which makes a free opening upward for the exit of pus. If the disease has progressed so far that suppuration is inevitable, it is better to change from cold to warm applications, and to change our internal remedies for hepar, merc., or silex. If the sac is very much swollen, and the skin over it has become thin, so that bursting is imminent, it is advisable to lay it open in a downward and slightly outward direction. If left to find its own way out, the matter may escape at some ulcerated portion of the sac, which permits it to flow beneath the adjoining cellular tissue, and thus create additional swellings, and finally find its way through the skin at considerable distance from its original seat. Our object should be to prevent complications of this kind, and to give the freest and speediest exit to the pus. After opening, the lips of the wound should be kept apart by a bit of lint to permit of free discharge, and the swelling poulticed if necessary. After a few days, when the inflammation has subsided, the canaliculus should be opened, and a probe passed into the sac to afford a free entrance and exit for the tears. The external opening of the sac may then be allowed to close.

If a considerable discharge of muco-purulent matter continues, the sac and duct may be syringed out with cold water daily, or with a solution of two grains of alum to the ounce of water. I have seen excellent results from using a grain or two of sul. of zinc to the ounce of water, administering at the same time zinc, or sul. of zinc, internally. I have used also to advantage a few drops to the ounce of water of tinct. of sanguinaria in conjunction with the administration of sang., internally. Generally speaking, however, vegetable solutions are in these cases less useful than mineral, in my experience. The solutions are to be employed daily, or every other day. To syringe the sac thoroughly, it is sometimes requisite to pass a cannula quite into it, attaching the syringe to the mouth of the cannula afterwards. If necessary to the introduction of the cannula, which is perhaps as large as a number four to six of the Bowman probe, the neck of the sac and the internal palpebral ligament may be incised with a probe-pointed knife.

The selection of internal remedies is very much controlled by the general condition of the patient and by the diathesis. In scrofulous subjects, for instance, merc., hepar, and calc. seem to be especially suitable, and will be indicated sometimes by the general symptoms. I have also used, with benefit, for such cases, kalihydriod., injecting daily the same, of the strength of one to three grains of the salt to an ounce of water. In other instances, macrot., stilling., and hydras., often selected for symptoms but remotely connected with the disease in question, have been serviceable. In acute and subacute cases, if the discharge is copious and purulent, no remedy compares for promptness and certainty of action with arg. nit., externally and internally, while in older or different cases, when the discharge is scantier and thinner, cup. sulph., externally and internally, is better. The injections of these salts should be commenced very cautiously, with a solution of not more than a grain to the ounce of water, and then, if necessary, later, the strength of the solution may be increased. The alum and the sul. of zinc are better when the discharge is more mucous in character, but very often in these lighter cases injections of cold water will be sufficient, in conjunction with internal remedies. In chronic cases, unless very mild, and of periodical recurrence, when internal remedies are curative through the restoration of the general health, mechanical means will be necessary as auxiliaries.

DILATATION OF THE SAC FROM DISEASE.

Firm pressure upon the sac will hasten its reduction to the normal size and condition. This can be made by a thick compress held in its place by a bandage. In chronic dilatation of the sac, where it is desired to apply the pressure for a considerable period, it will be found more convenient to use a small spring truss, attached to a narrow band passing around the head horizontally just over the eyes, and kept in place by another band running over the head at right angles to it.

FISTULA OF THE SAC.

In old cases where the bursting of the sac has occurred, or repeatedly occurred, a fistulous opening through the skin remains; and by this channel the tears flow over the cheek. In these cases an exit for the tears should be made by dilating the passage from above. The fistula will then heal of itself, or healing may be hastened by touching the edges of the opening with a crayon of mild nitrate of silver, or sulphate of copper. In cases of this kind, disease of the bone is sometimes present, and treatment, if undertaken at all, is often unsatisfactory.

CHRONIC CATARRH, OR BLENNORRHÆA OF THE LACHRYMAL PASSAGES,

May result from an acute inflammation of the sac; it may be merely an extension of a nasal catarrh, a catarrhal or granular ophthalmia, but much oftener, in my experience, it appears to be an idiopathic disease which comes on slowly and insidiously. A patient presents himself to be cured of "watering" of an eye. He will hardly be able to inform us accurately of the date of the commencement of his trouble. It was first noticed in cold weather, and especially when out in cold winds. Afterwards, it was annoying in-doors, occasionally, and now the "watering" of the eye is continuous. We diagnose the case at once by putting a finger over the lachrymal sac and pressing gently upwards, when a muco-serous discharge wells out through the punctum. It may be possible at this stage of the affection to press the contents downward through the nose. However this may be, if the patient is willing to give himself the trouble to press out the contents of the sac *sev-*

eral times a day, avoid cold winds, over-exertion of the eyes, and pay proper attention to the condition of his general health, the chances are that he may go on for years, and perhaps for a lifetime, without any increase of the disorder. In addition to these hygienic regulations, mild collyria of zinc or alum dropped into the inner corner of the eye with zincum or aluminum, internally, will often prove greatly beneficial. Furthermore, when the general health is at fault, one may frequently remove the lachrymal disorder by restoring the system to a healthy state.

TREATMENT BY PROBING.

Patients are frequently impatient under the above treatment, and unwilling generally to follow such strict hygienic rules; they desire a treatment of some definite duration, and which offers at the same time a tolerable chance of permanent cure. We then proceed to the removal of the stricture or strictures of the duct by probing. The probes used are usually of silver wire of uniform size throughout, like Bowman's, or they may be made with a bulb at the extremity, and flexible or elastic, like those called here the Williams probe. The Bowman probes are numbered from one to six or eight, No. 1 being quite fine, and No. 8 about $\frac{1}{16}$ of an inch in diameter. I generally commence with No. 2, and rarely go beyond

No. 4 or 5, in size. The probes are flexible, and will remain bent in any direction we may desire. Generally, the probe finds its way into the duct more readily if bent slightly at the end before introducing. In probing the left duct, we stand before the patient, and keeping the concavity of the bent probe always towards us, enter the canaliculus, which has previously been slit up, passing the probe in a horizontal direction, inclined slightly upward, at the same time stretching the integuments of the lower lid outward. Having reached the sac, as determined by the firm resistance of its inner wall to the end of the probe, and by the observation that the integuments at the inner angle of the eye do not appear to resist the probe or move forward with it, we turn the instrument in a vertical direction, and pass it down into the sac. To find and enter the nasal duct readily, the direction of the probe will now require to be slightly changed, so that its extremity shall point a little outward and forward, and, having entered the duct, it is to be pressed gently downward to the floor of the nose. If operating on the right lachrymal passage, we may hold the probe in the left hand, or, stand behind the patient, and use the right hand.

Probes of whalebone, gutta-percha, or laminaria digitata, a species of sea-weed, are sometimes used. The latter imbibe the moisture of the parts, and swell up to double, and sometimes treble, their original size when introduced.

A stricture may be situated at any point of the passage. Its most frequent seat is where the canaliculi join the sac, or below, where the latter is narrowed into the nasal duct. It is to be overcome by firm, but gradual and gentle, pressure downward. Frequently a change from a larger to a smaller probe will be successful. Generally, however, the larger one is to be preferred if much pressure is necessary, as less likely to lacerate the lining membrane. Tact, gentleness, and sometimes a good deal of perseverance, are necessary. One may sometimes try for two or three weeks, at intervals of two or three days, before overcoming a stricture. When we find it impossible to enter the sac from the lower canaliculus, we may succeed, perhaps, from the upper, or it may be necessary to divide the stricture before the probe can be introduced, with a narrow bistoury. Weber's delicate probe-pointed knife, or the narrow knife of Stilling, are suitable. The conical probe of Weber, which increases rapidly in size from the point, may often be used as a dilator to advantage, and the use of the knife be dispensed with. Occasionally, the lining of the sac is so much thickened from inflammation and swelling, that it seems impossible to find the entrance of the nasal duct from the sac. In such instances, we may do better to relinquish all attempts at probing until time and the employment of local and constitutional remedies have reduced the inflammation somewhat, when the probing may be again attempted with better chances of success. Having once succeeded, the operation should be repeated on every second or third day, gradually increasing the size of the probe, and gradually increasing the length of the intervals between each operation, until the flow of tears through the passage is unimpeded, and the secretion becomes normal in quantity and appearance.

THE USE OF THE STYLE.

Attempts have been made, and apparently with considerable success, to obviate the necessity for repeated probing, by the use of styles. Unlike the old-fashioned ones, these styles are introduced, like the probes, from above, and are to be used for some months. When the discharge is not great they may be worn days or weeks without changing, and it is claimed that the irritation set up when the style is first attempted to be worn soon passes off, and the patient finds it comfortable. They are made of silver or lead of different sizes, and may be flattened at the upper end so as to be bent over the lower lid like a hook. Where there is difficulty in keeping up the dilation of the strictured portion of the passage, and frequent relapses occur, it would seem that this method offers a chance of a permanent cure. It is said also to be available in cases where frequent visits to the surgeon are impossible. The styles are of wire, from $\frac{1}{24}$ to $\frac{1}{12}$ of an inch or more in diameter, and one and three-quarters if for the lower, or two inches in length, if intended for the upper canaliculus.

METHOD OF STILLING.

The new method of Stilling proposes to cure the disease radically by a single operation. He first finds the seat of the stricture by probing, and then withdrawing the probe, introduces a small narrow knife in its place, and incises the stricture in three or four different directions. This, according to the author, and others who have practised his method, is sufficient for a permanent cure, even in very severe cases. The *rationale* of this treatment is not very apparent. If it prove as successful as represented, it will be a welcome resource in obstinate cases, even if too severe a procedure for ordinary practice.

GENERAL REMARKS.

The most frequent obstacle to the permanant cure of catarrh or blennorrhœa is the tendency of the lachrymal passage to close again after it has been sucessfully dilated. I believe this tendency may be best overcome by a moderate and gentle dilation of the passages, and, when possible, avoiding all bruising, lacerating, and even cutting, of the lining membrane, and then by constitutional and local remedies, endeavoring to restore the diseased mucous surface to as healthy a condition as possible. Professor Arlt, of Vienna, rarely goes beyond the No. 4 Bowman probe, in size. He prefers not to risk a rupture of the epithelial lining of the passage, and remarks that at its nasal portion its normal capacity is not much greater than a No. 4 probe, and that where the canaliculi join the sac the diameter is less than that of No. 5. The following is his measurement on the cadavre of the sac and duct. A millimetre is equal to about two-fifths of a line:—

THE SAC.	THE NASAL DUCT.
Length, ten. Width, four. Antero-posterior diameter, two millimetres.	Length, about ten. Width and antero-pos. diam., each 1½ to 2½ millimetres.

In the zeal for dilating the duct as widely as possible, so as to prevent its reclosure, the catarrhal inflammation of the lining membrane and the dilatation of the sac are overlooked. The permeability of the tear passage, although a necessary stage in the progress of cure, does not always complete it. The abnormally dilated sac is to be reduced by pressure, and the catarrh treated by local and constitutional remedies, otherwise the germs of fresh inflammations are left behind, and the old obstruction reappears.

OTHER OPERATIVE MEASURES.

The operation for obliteration (so called) of the lachrymal sac by incision, and the application of caustics, or the actual cautery, has fallen nearly into disuse. The sac is rarely obliterated by the operation, and the result is generally unsatisfactory.

Herzenstein's operation for rupturing portions of the lachrymal passage does not seem to have met with favor as yet. The removal of the lachrymal gland, as practised by Mr. Laurence for severe cases of stillicidium, appears to promise more, but will very likely be found too severe an operation for private practice, unless in very exceptional cases.

THE LACHRYMAL GLAND.

The lachrymal gland is subject, in rare instances, to acute and chronic inflammations, hypertrophy, fistula, and to cystic formations. The acute and chronic inflammatory affections of this gland are amenable to such treatment as would be suitable for similar affections in other parts of the body. The disease of the gland is so rare that details of symptoms and treatment may be left for larger treatises.

In more than one hundred thousand cases of disease of the eye observed at the Ophthalmic Hospital in London, less than twenty cases of affections of this gland are recorded.

CHAPTER XVII.

AFFECTIONS OF THE WHOLE EYE AND OF THE ORBIT.

HYDROPHTHALMIA, KERATO-GLOBUS.

DROPSY of the eye (so called) affects principally the anterior half of the eyeball. The peculiar stare which the prominence of the eyes gives the patient is very striking. The corneæ are increased in size, the anterior chambers in depth, and the irides are tremulous for lack of support. The pupils are dilated, and sometimes pear-shaped, and ultimately vision is more or less impaired. The sclerotica grows thin and bluish as the disease progresses, and all parts of the eye are finally involved. The progress of the affection is usually slow. It is probably incurable. Remedies like arsen., merc., and those suitable for affections of the cornea generally, may be prescribed, in the hope, at least, of retarding the progress of the malady. Surgically, repeated paracentesis corneæ, and iridectomy have been productive of benefit.

EXOPHTHALMIC GOITRE, GRAVES' DISEASE,

As far as progressive bulging of the globe is concerned, resembles dropsy of the eye. It is associated with hypertrophy of the thyroid gland, palpitation of the heart, and subsequent dilatation of its cavities, anæmia, visceral derangements, and in females with amenorrhœa. The disease is also accompanied by great nervous excitement and a capricious temper. Its progress is slow, and the prognosis is not as uniformly unfavorable as in dropsy of the eye. The treatment cannot be laid down on account of the almost numberless complications which the disease may present, but I have no doubt that judicious homœopathic treatment would afford encouraging results. Hydropathic treatment is to be favorably mentioned as having been serviceable in this affection.

MEDULLARY CANCER OF THE EYE

Has been spoken of under the name of *glioma retinæ*. *Melanotic cancer* is probably the same disease, with the addition of more or less black pigment in its structure. *Sarcoma* is a recurrent growth, requiring similar treatment to cancer, but exhibits less tendency to secondary deposits. Before breaking through the anterior tunics of the eye, it has been mistaken for glaucoma. It can only be distinguished from cancer by microscopic examination. *Ophthalmitis*, or suppuration of the whole eye, is noticed in the chapter on the Choroid.

DISEASES OF THE ORBIT.

I have not the space to speak in detail of diseases of the orbit, and must refer the reader to works on general surgery. As regards diagnosis, tumors of the orbit are accompanied by more or less protrusion of the eye, and by diminished mobility of the globe, and sooner or later there is impaired vision. In inflammation and abscess of the cellular tissue there will be added to these symptoms pain in and around the ball, and tenderness on pressure of the globe backward. Tumors will generally require to be removed together with the eyeball, and inflammation and abscess will demand the same general treatment as if located elsewhere.

CHAPTER XVIII.

INJURIES OF THE EYE.

THE EYELIDS.

For contusions and ecchymoses of the eyelids we have excellent remedies in our arnica, hamamelis, and calendula. Lacerated or incised wounds are to be treated as usual in other parts of the body, except that especial care should be taken in accurately approximating the edges of such wounds in the lids, so as to guard against deformity. In burns and scalds, great care will be necessary during the cicatricial period to prevent plastic union of the two lids at the angles. This is to be prevented by inunction with simple cerate, and by directing that the lids be frequently opened. To prevent ectropium and a contraction which might prevent the eye from closing (lagophthalmos), the lids should be kept as much as possible on the stretch, and be bandaged with extreme care. For the same reasons it is always advisable, when possible, to bring the edges of wounds of the lids together by fine interrupted suture, rather than leave them to unite by granulation, and risk a loss of substance and contraction.

INJURIES OF THE CONJUNCTIVA,

Of a chemical nature, are quite common. Those from quick lime are of the most serious to which the eye is subject. Complete destruction of the tissues of the parts, with which the lime comes in contact, may result. Slaked lime, mortar, and plaster are not so rapidly destructive in their effect, but may in the end prove nearly as fatal. The chief danger, even in cases where the burn is not very extensive or very deep, is in loss of sight from opacity of the cornea. The whiteness of the corneal opacities in these cases is very marked, and it has been demonstrated, recently, that the cicatricial tissue reproduced after these injuries contains lime.

THE TREATMENT.

It is wiser not to attempt to neutralize the alkali by the use of weak acid. The eye is very intolerant of acids in these cases, and they can hardly be of service unless applied *immediately* after the accident. It is better therefore to resort to olive oil at once, a small quantity of which is to be dropped into the eye. The lids are then to be everted, and the loose particles of lime removed with a delicate spatula. If the epithelial layer of the cornea is destroyed it should be removed, and, if possible, the cauterized portions of the corneal substance should also be taken off, so that the reproduction of tissue may not only be speedy, but that the new tissue may be free from depositions of lime, and transparent. After the application of a few drops more of sweet oil, the lids should be closed, cold-water dressings used for the first few days, and acon. and arn. administered.

In injuries from strong acids, a solution of carb. of potash, or soda, five grains to an ounce of water, may be used at first if the eye is seen soon after the injury. When this is not convenient, warm water may be substituted. Olive oil should then be used. In burns and scalds of the conjunctiva from hot fluids, olive oil should also be applied, the lids closed, and the eye lightly bandaged, as directed in chapter second. Oil should be dropped into the eye two or three times a day, the lids cleansed from all discharge, and the bandage readjusted. Acon. and arn. will be the remedies indicated for internal use.

Injuries from gunpowder are sometimes serious, not only from the scorching and burning of the conjunctiva from the explosion, but from the circumstance also, that unexploded grains of the powder are deposited in and upon the conjunctiva, and are sometimes forced through it into the tissue of the sclerotic, and often imbedded in the substance of the cornea. The lids are to be everted and syringed so as to remove all loose powder, then all superficially imbedded grains in the conjunctiva and cornea are to be removed with the spatula or broad needle, and olive or castor oil dropped into the eye two or three times a day, and such general treatment resorted to as seems necessary.

Mechanical injuries of the conjunctiva, from foreign bodies such as cinders, dust, particles of iron, steel, glass, and the like, generally occasion a good deal of injection, and not unfrequently severe ciliary neuralgia, photophobia, and lachrymation. In the case of a single foreign body, like a cinder, it will generally be found beneath the upper lid, and sometimes far back in the retrotarsal region. A small spatula may be used to remove it. It is not worth while however for a surgeon to attempt to do this without everting the upper lid, nor by the introduction of other foreign bodies, like smooth pebbles called eye-stones, or smooth round seeds. Leave such proceedings as these to the foremen of establishments, and to domestic practitioners. The method of everting the upper lid is described elsewhere. A year or more ago a lady came to me for a conjunctivitis of one eye, accompanied by severe ciliary irritation, pain, and photophobia. She had been for three weeks under the treatment of a colleague, and during all this time she thought that she had not had one comfortable night's rest. Her symptoms all pointed to a foreign body, and on everting the upper lid, there laid partially imbedded in the substance of the conjunctiva, a minute bit of quartz with its sharp edges and angles. Its removal cured her at once. She had suffered for three weeks, when the exercise of a little circumspection would have relieved her at any time in three minutes. Splinters or other substances beneath the conjunctiva, if found impracticable to remove with delicate forceps, may be cut out with curved scissors. Impalpable particles of dust or sand may be washed out with the syringe and warm water.

In the "American Journal of the Medical Sciences," vol. 50, p. 561, among other cases of neglected foreign bodies in the eye, is that of a German who was treated some time for granulated lids, until finally the cause of the affection was discovered in a neglected "eye-stone" which he had put into his eye six months previously, and which he thought had dropped out while he was asleep, as his wife said she had seen it in the bed. The removal of the "eye-stone" cured the eye. In the "Ophthalmic Review," vol. I., p. 337, is related in full, the case of an old man who fell to the bottom of the stairs, and applied to a surgeon for a wound in the conjunctiva at the inner angle of the right eye. After a week's treatment the presence of a foreign body was suspected, and the next day a cast-iron hat-peg three and three-tenths inches in length was drawn from the wound. The patient, wonderful to relate, recovered without unfavorable symptoms. Small particles, like gravel or dust, are to be removed by everting the lids and syringing them, and also by the use of the spatula or blunt probe, when necessary.

ANCHYLOBLEPHARON

Is the union of the margin of the lids with each other, either directly or by membranous bands. It is a result of injury, or ulceration from disease. The union is to be severed with the scissors or the scalpel, and reunion prevented by frequent separation, and by anointing the cut surfaces with olive oil.

SYMBLEPHARON

Is the union of the inner surface of the lids with the eyeball, and may also be direct and close, or by membranous bands. In the latter case, the bands of union may be divided, and daily dressing with olive oil may possibly prevent a reunion. Generally however, and especially when the adhesions are at all extensive, reunion after separation cannot be prevented, and all attempts of whatever nature are fruitless. The condition is irremediable. The cause of the affection is an injury, usually a burn from hot fluid, metal, lime, or mortar.

DIAGNOSIS AND TREATMENT OF FOREIGN BODIES WITHIN THE GLOBE.

The diagnosis is sometimes quite difficult. When the foreign body cannot be seen, with or without the aid of lateral illumination and the ophthalmoscope, we may suspect its presence;

If the pain does not yield to the usual palliative treatment, and is apparently disproportionate to the visible inflammation.

If the inflammation does not appear to be controlled by the treatment, to the usual extent.

If symptoms of inflammation of the deeper structures of the eye are present.

If there is a circumscribed iritis with exudation, limited to a given point, no foreign body being visible, the eye having been struck by a splinter of metal. I recall a case like this in the clinic of Professor Graefe, where he made an iridectomy, and then removed the invisible bit of metal from behind the iris.

If there is non-union, or only partial union, of a wound through which a foreign body may have entered the eye.

In cases like the above, where the irritation or

inflammation is continuous, an attempt should be made to find and remove the foreign body, and failing in this, the eye should be removed. Where the foreign body can be seen, it should be removed in all cases when it can be done without serious risk of loss of the eye. It must be extracted at any hazard to the eye, if irritation, pain, and inflammation, are engendered by its presence, lest sympathetic inflammation destroy the other eye. Inflammation recurring in an eye which has lost all visual power from former injury, whether the presence of a foreign body be suspected or not, demands the removal of the eye. When a foreign body, like a bit of percussion cap for instance, remains in the eye, but causes no irritation, the sight of the eye being unimpaired by it, and its extraction would be hazardous to the eye, it may be left in its place; but the patient should be enlightened as to the nature of the risk he is taking, and be instructed to return to the surgeon the moment symptoms of irritation come on in the injured eye. The insertion of an artificial eye after the operation of enucleation *for sympathetic ophthalmia*, should be deferred for a number of months after all irritation in the remaining eye has disappeared. This extreme caution is necessary, lest symptoms of irritation be reawakened by the presence of the artificial eye.

THE CORNEA.

Injuries of the cornea are more to be feared than those of the conjunctiva, from the fact that opacities upon its surface impair vision. Fragments of metals, or splinters, in its substance, occasion great ciliary irritation, pain, injection, photophobia, and lachrymation. If the foreign body, owing to its small size or color, is difficult of detection, the pupil may be dilated with atropine so as to enlarge the dark background, and then oblique illumination and a magnifying glass employed. A delicate spatula or broad needle may be used for removing the foreign substance, and in unruly or very nervous subjects, it may be necessary to fix the eye with forceps. This is not usually necessary; but the operation of removing substances imbedded in the cornea is one of considerable delicacy, and sometimes requires a good deal of quickness and dexterity. Chemical injuries of the cornea may be treated as directed under Injuries of the Conjunctiva. Clear cuts, or punctures of the cornea, heal readily, and generally leave no scar behind. The danger in these cases lies in the possibility that the iris or the lens may have been wounded, and iritis or cataract supervene. The treatment of wounds or injuries of the cornea requires entire rest of the eyes, and the administration of acon. or arn.; if the ciliary neuralgia be considerable, cham., spig., or macrot., warm fomentations and the instillation of atropine, as palliatives, may be required. Olive oil or castor oil is very grateful to the eye after the removal of a foreign body, and in abrasions of the epithelial surface of the cornea, and the simple bandage described in the second chapter of this work should be applied.

THE IRIS AND LENS.

If a wound of the iris is clean, with no laceration, it may heal at once without iritis or suppuration. If a bit of iris protrude through an opening in the cornea, and cannot be readily replaced, either by careful manipulation, or the employment of atropine or calabar bean, it may be excised. Foreign bodies, such as bits of percussion cap, or steel, remaining in the substance of the iris, will almost invariably set up an iritis, and should therefore be removed by an iridectomy, excising that portion of the iris in which the foreign body is situated. Injuries of the cornea and iris, like other injuries, sometimes result much less disastrously than we have reason to predict. I recall the case of a child two years old, that had run a blade of a pair of scissors into the right eye towards the inner angle, penetrating the cornea and iris. I expected of course, traumatic cataract, but the direction of the instrument was such that the capsule of the lens was left intact. Iritis ensued, yet, the eye finally recovered perfectly, leaving no corneal opacity behind, and no deformity, except a slight displacement of the pupil from a small synechia posterior, at the point of perforation of the iris. In all wounds, when the anterior or posterior chamber has been entered, the eye should be bandaged immediately.

Hemorrhage into the anterior chamber may result from a wound of the iris, or from a detachment of its ciliary border. It may be so extensive as to completely hide the pupil and iris from view. I have known it to occur to this extent in the operation of iridectomy. It is the least dangerous form of intra-ocular hemorrhage, and the blood is usually soon absorbed. A fold of linen wet from time to time with a lotion of ten drops of tinc. ham. to the ounce of cold water, should be laid over the closed lids, and a simple bandage applied.

When a wound of the anterior chamber is large, and the iris bulges, forming a sac distended with aqueous humor, it is not safe to excise it lest a further prolapse occur. It should be pricked at intervals, with a fine needle, so as to cause it to dwindle, and permit the edges of the wound to approximate. Later, it can be excised, if necessary. Traumatic cataract has been already spoken of.

THE SCLEROTICA.

Incised wounds in the sclera are not usually dangerous unless very extensive, but do not heal as readily as wounds in the substance of the cornea. Care must therefore be taken that the edges of the cut approximate exactly, and, if necessary to this end, a fine suture may be employed. *Rupture of the sclerotic* is a far more dangerous accident, frequently involving dislocation of the lens, prolapse of the iris, great loss of vitreous and internal hemorrhage of the eye. Soothing applications should be made, and if after a few days no perception of light return, it is better and safer to enucleate the injured globe. *Injuries in the ciliary region* are chiefly dangerous as giving rise to sympathetic ophthalmia.

SYMPATHETIC OPHTHALMIA

Is the name given to the inflammation set up in the sound eye as a result of injury to its fellow eye. Injuries in the ciliary region, with loss of vitreous and wounding of the lens, are the most frequent cause. Foreign bodies remaining within the eye are also a frequent cause, and although such bodies may not give rise to irritation in the wounded eye for many years, where once the irritation occurs, sympathetic ophthalmia in the other eye is often the result.

Sympathetic disease is never to be considered as impossible so long as there is tenderness of the injured eye to touch in the ciliary region.

The nature of sympathetic ophthalmia is that of a malignant and destructive iritis, which spreads rapidly to the ciliary body and the choroid. In the beginning there is irritation, some injection of the conjunctiva, photophobia, lachrymation, increased tension, and severe asthenopic symptoms quickly supervening upon any attempt to use the eyes for reading, or for any similar purpose. At this stage of the affection there is no pain when the eyes are at rest; later, there is some supraorbital neuralgia, iritis, great effusion of lymph, adhesion between the iris and anterior capsule, the choroid and vitreous become involved, and atrophy of the latter is followed by softening of the globe.

ENUCLEATION OF THE INJURED EYE.

The only justifiable course to pursue when sympathetic ophthalmia is once begun in the uninjured eye is to remove the injured one at once. Enucleation of the ball, under complete etherization of the patient is not a formidable procedure. The lids are to be well separated by a speculum; one or two assistants with sponges should be near to remove the blood during the operation, so that the view of the operator may be as little obstructed as possible. Suppose the left eye to be removed. The operator stands in front of the patient, who lies on a couch. Seizing the conjunctiva at the outer side of the globe near the insertion of the rectus externus, with the forceps, he makes an incision, and carries his blunt-pointed scissors quite around the circle of the cornea, dividing the conjunctiva as near the corneal limbus as possible. He then inserts a blade of the curved scissors beneath the external rectus, and divides it close to its sclerotic insertion. Relinquishing now his first hold with the forceps, he seizes the globe at the point of insertion of the rectus muscle, just divided, in order to obtain a firmer hold, so as to move the eyeball at will. The superior and inferior recti and oblique muscles are successively divided with the scissors close to the ball, and then with larger scissors, the globe being pulled as far forward and towards the nasal side as possible, the optic nerve is cut: a gush of blood follows from the ophthalmic artery, the forceps are relinquished, the ball is grasped with the fingers, the rectus internus divided, and the enucleation is completed. The hemorrhage is trivial, and readily controlled by cold water. In case of encephaloid of the globe, or tumors of the orbit, and like cases, the difficulties of the operation are much increased, and the various steps in it will be different, and other instruments may be necessary.

WHEN TO REMOVE THE INJURED EYE.

How soon, after the first symptoms of sympathetic irritation manifest themselves in the sound eye, shall the injured one be removed? Inasmuch as symptoms of irritation do not always give rise to the disease, and as the disease if it occur, is not absolutely certain to be of that fatal type which ends in destruction of the eye, and the total blindness of our patient, how long may we wait with safety? This question is sometimes difficult to answer; but in case the injured eye is already blind, or all hope of restoration of vision lost, we need not wait at all, for in such an event its removal is in no respect contra-indicated, and will in all instances guarantee the integrity of the remaining eye, *provided no symptoms of sympathetic ophthalmia have yet made their appearance.* After sympathetic disease has once commenced in the uninjured eye, the removal of the other is not a certain, although the best, remedy known, and succeeds in saving the remaining eye, especially if done at an early stage of the disease, in a vast majority of cases. Another means, that of division of the ciliary muscle, has recently been practised with some success. It might be worth while to try this, provided tolerable sight in the injured eye were still probable. An incision in the conjunctiva at that point in the ciliary region, which is sensitive to the touch, is made with the forceps and scissors. The eye being steadied, a puncture is made in the sclerotica over the ciliary muscle, with a cataract knife, and the wound is closed with a suture.

The general treatment should enforce the strictest hygienic regulations, absolute rest of the eyes, a subdued light at home, and the protection of dark glasses out of doors. The diet should be nutritious and generous. The pupil should be kept dilated *ad maximum*, and internal and other remedies, such as recommended for iritis, are to be used.

A CASE OF INJURY OF THE EYE.

I have a patient at the present time, a farmer, aged seventy, who in chopping wood was struck on the eye by a chip. I saw him the next day. He was suffering severely from ciliary neuralgia. No wound or bruise of the cornea or sclerotic was observable. Vision was so much impaired that only night from day could be distinguished. The iris was completely paralyzed by the shock, the pupil dilated and immovable. Ophthalmoscopic symptoms negative from cloudiness of the vitreous humor. After a few days, under the internal administration of bell. and spig., and the external use of arn., warm fomentations, and atropine instillations, the pain subsided, and the eye felt comparatively comfortable. Soreness of the ball remained, and remains still. There was a mere perception of light in the eye, and no more. At one time, about three weeks after the injury, the sight improved so that large objects could be discerned; it then gradually failed, and is now wholly gone. The eye has not been removed for these reasons.

Although there is considerable pain, photophobia, and lachrymation, at times, in the sound eye, as well as in the injured one, I find that it never occurs spontaneously, but only after work in the fields, or from other occupation requiring a stooping position.

The patient is seventy years old, and the probability of the occurrence of sympathetic ophthalmia is much less in aged than in youthful subjects. He lives near, and can remain under my immediate supervision. These circumstances determined me to wait and operate only when the first threatening symptoms of sympathetic disease in the sound eye should appear. A year has now elapsed, the eyes are still irritable, permit of little use for near objects, but, on the whole, there is a steady improvement.

SYMPATHETIC IRRITATION,

In the uninjured eye, may occur without giving rise to ophthalmia. It may be recurrent, coming on whenever there is an exacerbation of the inflammation in the injured eye, but it is to be distinguished from sympathetic ophthalmia by the important fact that no iritis with effusion of lymph is present. There is some injection, lachrymation, ciliary neuralgia, and severe asthenopic symptoms whenever use of the eye is attempted. Removal of the injured eye cures sympathetic irritation at once. When this operation, or division of the ciliary muscle, is not resorted to, measures directed to the improvement of the injured eye, through internal medication, soothing applications, and strict hygienic precautions, may be tried.

CHAPTER XIX.

LIST OF A FEW INTERNAL REMEDIES WITH THE OPHTHALMIC AFFECTIONS, OR THE SUBJECTIVE AND OBJECTIVE SYMPTOMS OF THE EYES, FOR WHICH THEY HAVE BEEN FOUND USEFUL IN MY PRACTICE.

THE list which follows comprises merely the remedies which have been administered from indications furnished by the eye alone. Others have been found useful also, but they have been selected on account of symptoms apart from those of the eye, and such as are familiar to all general practitioners. Many remedies having a strong affinity for the eye, judged by their pathogenesis, have not, in my experience, been found reliable. The diseases or symptoms given below have been repeatedly cured or relieved by a single remedy, the name of which is placed opposite each group. The dilutions or triturations used were the first, second, or third.

ACONITE. — In the early stage of inflammations of the conjunctiva, cornea, and iris, and after surgical operations.

ALUMINA. — In chronic blepharitis of adults, and in blennorrhœa of the lachrymal passage, with thin discharge.

ARG. NIT. — In affections of the lining membrane of the lids, and of the lachrymal duct and sac when there is a copious discharge of pus.

ARNICA. — In injuries, and in hemorrhage beneath the conjunctiva.

ARSENICUM. — In superficial and deep-seated ulceration of the cornea, especially in scrofulous subjects. Catarrhal oph., with thin secretion and irritation of the edges of the lids. Ulceration of the tarsal edges, with thin secretion.

BAPTISIA. — In mild purulent ophthalmia (puls.).

BELLADONNA. — In photophobia; injection of the ocular conjunctiva; congestion of the retina and optic nerve; dilation of the pupil; ciliary neuralgia and pain in the optic nerve, with congestion. Neuritis optica (diagnosed with the ophthalmoscope).

CONIUM. — Photophobia in scrofulous subjects or in scrofulous ophthalmia (tart. emet.).

BRYONIA. — Scleritis or episcleritis. Conjunctivitis with soreness of the eyeballs to the touch and on moving them (sang.).

CACTUS. — Hyperæmia of retina and optic nerve; optic neuritis. Asthenopic symptoms in conjunction with a tendency to congestive headache or flushed face.

CHAMOMILLA. — Ciliary neuralgia, especially in scrof. or purulent ophthalmia of children (spigel. bell.).

CUPRUM AND CUP. SULPH. — In chronic ophthalmiæ, with rather scanty mixed discharge of pus and mucus.

EUPHRASIA. — Simple or catarrhal conjunctivitis, with copious secretion or lachrymation (puls.).

GELSEMINUM. — Accommodative asthenopia, with the usual subjective symptoms. Diplopia (from functional disturbance of accommodation in one eye). Ptosis from partial paralysis. Chronic spasms of the orbicularis. Nictitation. Hyperæsthesia retinæ, with photophobia (nux v.).

GLONOINE. — Venous hyperæmia, or congestion of the retina and optic nerve (cactus, phosph, sang.).

GRAPHITES. — Blepharitis, with pustular eruption along the tarsi and loss of cilia (hepar).

HAMAMELIS. — Redness of the conjunctiva and asthenopic symptoms. Hemorrhage into the ant. chamber. Bruises of the lids. (To be used externally at the same time in each of the above.)

HEPAR. — Purulent ophthal. with merc. Inveterate blepharitis with purulent secretion, in scrofulous subjects. Chronic corneitis.

HYDRASTIN. — In acutè catarrhal ophthalmiæ, with profuse discharge, especially in scrofulous or ill-nourished subjects.

KALI HYD. — Inflam. of lach. sac, with mucous discharge. Syphilitic iritis, choroiditis, and corneitis

LEPTAND. — Asthenopic symptoms, with yellow look of the sclerotica.

MACROTIN. — Accommodative, retinal, and muscular asthenopia. Photophobia from asthenopia; hyperæmia of conjunctiva, iris, choroid, and retina, due to prolonged exertion of myopic or hypermetropic eyes. Soreness of the eyeball to touch and on moving it (bry.). Aching pain in the eye (spig. merc.).

MERC. — Blepharitis, chronic or otherwise; meibomian cysts; purulent ophthal. with copious discharge; corneitis diffusa, superficial and deep-seated ulceration of the cornea; pustular ophthalmia; syphilitic disease of any or all the different structures of the eye; episcleritis; pain in the eyeball at night; scrofulous ophthalmia, with photophobia.

NUX V. — Asthenopic symptoms. Photophobia from retinal hyperæsthesia. Dilatation of the pupil from spinal irritation. Diplopia from muscular asthenopia, from paralytic strabismus. Paralysis of sixth nerve (rectus externus). Homonymous diplopia. Weakened power of accommodation in one eye from over-exerting it. Severe pain in the eyes, and during the night, with conjunctival injection, brought on by overuse of the eyes, especially by artificial light (gels. merc.). Spasmodic or involuntary closure of the eyes in adults (gels.).

OPIUM. — Hyperæmia of the conjunctiva and borders of the tarsi, with injection of the ocular conjunctiva in connection with congestive headache.

PULS. — Catarrhal ophthalmia with mucous secretion. Styes, especially in children and at the age of pubescence.

PHOSPH. — Retinal hyperæmia with congestion to the head. Flashes of light, dazzling points, or rings of various colors, before the eyes, indicating extreme sensitiveness of the retina.

SANG. — Retinal congestions, with tendency to flushed face and congestive headaches. Superficial injection of the eyeball, with feeling of soreness.

SCUTEL. — Spasmodic twitchings of the lids.

Sepia. — Acne ciliaris.

Spigelia. — Conjunctivitis and iritis in children, particularly in those of scrofulous diathesis. Congestion of the ciliary vessels, as indicated by the pinkish zone around the cornea. Severe pain in and around the eyes, and on moving them. Severe photophobia from ciliary nervous irritation.

Staphysagria. — In hordeolum, to prevent recurrence.

Sulphur. — In chronic ophthalmia scrofulosa, with superficial corneitis, the pinkish zone well marked around the edge of the cornea, and photophobia (merc. spigel.).

Tart. emet. — Photophobia in scrofulous ophthalmia of children. Pustular conjunctivitis.

Zincum. — Acute retinitis albumenurica.

Zinc. sul. — Conjunctivitis, simple, catarrhal, and mild purulent, when the discharge is not very copious. Catarrh of the lachrymal passages.

CHAPTER XX.

TEST TYPE.

THE first series of test type is presented merely as a convenience in noting the state of the vision, with or without glasses, for reading or near objects. The different sized print is numbered, so that a record can be made from time to time, and the progressive improvement or failure in visual power accurately determined. The second series, made up of different sized gothic letters, is intended for the more exact measurement of the patient's acuteness of vision. The numbers in this series indicate the distance at which an emmetropic eye should distinguish the letters. The letters of No. 6 should be named readily, in a good light, at six feet, 10 at ten feet, 20 at twenty feet, and so on. If No. 20 can be seen only as far as ten feet, then $V=\frac{10}{20}$ or $\frac{1}{2}$; if it can be seen at twenty feet, then $V=1$, and the eye is emmetropic. Occasionally a person will be met with who can read the letters at a much greater distance than the average. I have met those who could read Snellen No. 6 quite easily at ten feet, but such instances are not common. In experimenting, however, with a considerable number of persons, I have found it desirable, practically, to place the standard of normal vision considerably higher than Jaeger, and somewhat higher than Snellen.

FIRST SERIES.

No. 1.

I think it does not matter just when I first came to Venice. Yesterday and to-day are the same here. I arrived one winter morning about five o'clock, and was not so full of Soul as I might have been in warmer weather. Yet I was resolved not to go to my hotel in the omnibus (the large, many-seated boat so-called), but to have a gondola solely for myself and my luggage. The porter who seized my valise in the station, inferred from some very polyglottic Italian of mine the nature of my wish, and ran out and threw that slender piece of luggage into a gondola. I followed, lighted to my seat by a beggar in picturesque and desultory costume. He was one of a class of mendicants whom I came, for my sins, to know better in Venice, and whom I dare say every traveller

No. 2.

recollects – the merciless tribe who hold your gondola to shore, and affect to do you a service and not a displeasure, and pretend not to be abandoned swindlers. The Venetians call them *gransieri*, or crab-catchers; but as yet I did not know the name or the purpose of this *poverino*, at the station, but merely saw that he had the Venetian eye for color: in the distribution and arrangement of his fragments of dress he had produced some miraculous effects of red, and he was altogether as infamous a figure as any friend of brigands would like to meet in a lonely place. He did not offer to stab me and sink my body in the Grand Canal, as, in all Venetian

No. 3.

keeping, I felt that he ought to have done; but he implored an alms, and I hardly know now whether to exult or regret that I did not understand him, and left him empty-handed. I suppose that he withdrew again the blessings which he advanced me, as we pushed out into the canal: but I heard nothing, for the wonder of Venice was already upon me. All my nether-spirit, so to speak, was dulled and jaded with the long, cold, railway journey from Vienna, while every surface-sense was taken and tangled in the bewildering brilliancy and novelty of Venice. For I

No. 4.

think there can be nothing else in the world so full of glittering and exquisite surprise, as that first glimpse of Venice which the traveller catches as he issues from the railway station by night, and looks upon her peerless strangeness. There is something in the blessed breath of Italy (how quickly, coming south, you know it, and how bland it is, after the harsh, transalpine air!) which prepares you for your nocturnal advent into Venice; and O you! whoever you are, that journey toward this enchanted city for the first time, let me tell you how happy I count

No. 5.

you! There lies before you for your pleasure, the spectacle of such singular beauty as no picture can ever show you nor book tell you; beauty which you shall feel perfectly but once, and regret for ever.

For my own part, as the gondola slipped away from the blaze and bustle of the station down the gloom and silence of the broad canal, I forgot that I had been freezing two days and nights; that I was at that moment very cold and a little homesick. I could at first feel nothing

No. 6.

but that beautiful silence, broken only by the star-silvered dip of the oars. Then on either hand I saw stately palaces rise gray and lofty from the dark waters, holding here and there a lamp against their faces, which brought balconies, and columns, and carven arches into momentary relief, and threw long streams of crimson into the canal. I could see by that uncertain glimmer how fair

No. 7.

was all, but not how sad and old: and so unhaunted by any pang for the decay that afterwards saddened me amid the forlorn beauty of Venice, I glided on. I have no doubt it was a proper time to think all the fantastic things in the world, and I thought them; but they passed vaguely through my mind, without at all interrupting the sensations of sight and sound. Indeed, the past and present mixed there, and the moral and

No. 8.

material were blent in the sentiment of utter novelty and surprise. The quick boat slid through old troubles of mine, and unlooked-for events gave it the impulse that carried it beyond, and safely around sharp corners of life. And all the while I knew that this was a progress through narrow and crooked canals, and past marble angles of palaces. But I did not know then that this fine confusion

No. 9.

of sense and spirit was the first faint perception of the charm of life in Venice.

Dark, funereal barges like my own had flitted by, and the gondoliers had warned each other at every turning with hoarse, lugubrious cries; the lines of balconied palaces had never ended; — here and there at their doors larger craft were moored, with

No. 10.

dim figures of men moving uncertainly about on them. At last we had passed abruptly out of the Grand Canal into one of the smaller channels, and from comparative light into a darkness only remotely affected by some far-streaming corner lamp. But always the pallid, stately palaces; always the dark heaven with

No. 11.

its trembling stars above, and the dark water with its trembling stars below; but now innumerable bridges, and an utter lonesomeness, and ceaseless sudden turns and windings. One could not resist a vague feeling of anxiety, in these

No. 12.

strait and solitary passages, which was part of the strange enjoyment of the time, and which was referable to the novelty, the hush, the darkness, and the

No. 13.

piratical appearance and unaccountable pauses of the gondoliers. Was not this Venice, and is not Venice for ever associ-

No. 14.

ated with bravoes and unexpected dagger-thrusts? That valise of mine might represent

No. 15.

unbounded wealth to the uncultivated eye.

No. 16.

Who, if I made an out cry, could understand the Facts of the Situa tion, as we say in the journals ? To move on

[HOWELLS' VENETIAN LIFE.

SECOND SERIES.

No. 2.

LHDETFCIUO

No. 3.

E U C F O P G T H L

No. 5.

G T O H L E Q F D I

No. 6.

H G F D P U O I E

No. 8.

I G O T C L E F U

No. 10.

U F T D H G P O E

No. 12.

Q E C P U F D I L

No. 14.

P D L F H O T G I

No. 20.

F P L O H

No. 32.

F H G T

No. 50.

U C P

No. 70.

No. 100.

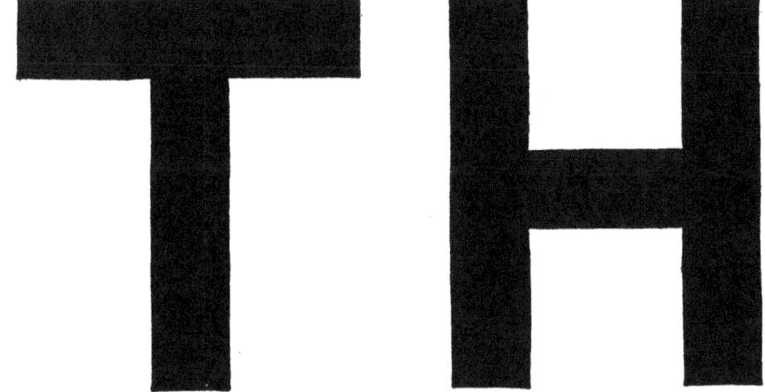

No. 200.

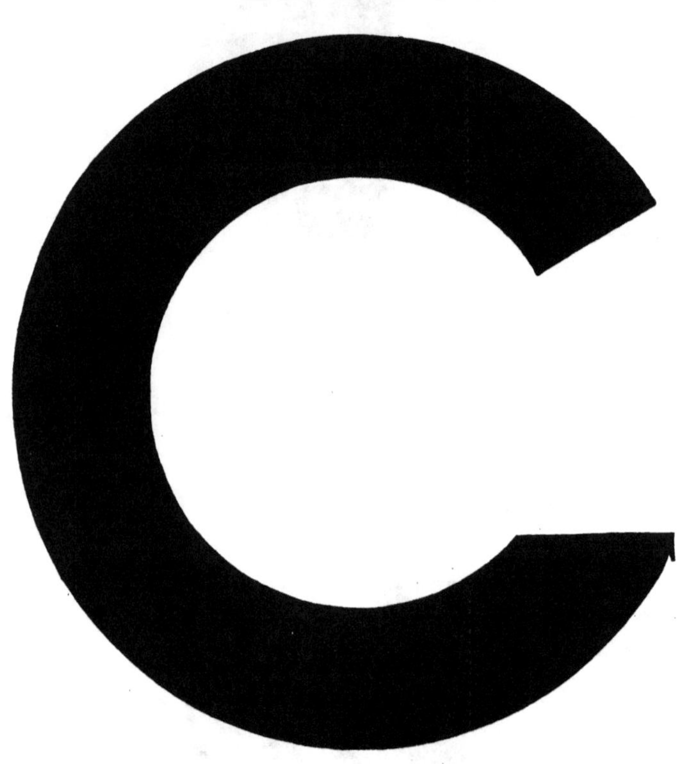

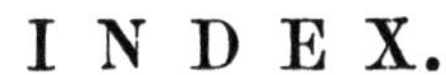

INDEX.

INDEX.

Cambridge: Stereotyped and Printed by John Wilson and Son.

www.ingramcontent.com/pod-product-compliance
Lightning Source LLC
LaVergne TN
LVHW010206110826
845151LV00002B/616

* 9 7 8 1 4 2 5 5 3 7 3 0 2 *